DISCLAIMER AND TERMS OF USE AGREEMENT:

(Please Read This Before Using This Report)

This information is not presented by a medical practitioner and is for educational and informational purposes only. The content is not intended to be a substitute for professional medical advice, diagnosis, or treatment. Always seek the advice of your physician or other qualified health provider with any questions you may have regarding a medical condition. Never disregard professional medical advice or delay in seeking it because of something you have read.

Since natural and/or dietary supplements are not FDA approved, they must be accompanied by a two-part disclaimer on the product label: that the statement has not been evaluated by FDA and that the product is not intended to "diagnose, treat, cure or prevent any disease.

The author and publisher of this course and the accompanying materials have used their best efforts in preparing this course. The author and publisher make no representation or warranties with respect to the accuracy, applicability, fitness, or completeness of the contents of this course. The information contained in this course is strictly for educational purposes. Therefore, if you wish to apply ideas contained in this course, you are taking full responsibility for your actions.

The author and publisher disclaim any warranties (express or implied), merchantability, or fitness for any particular purpose. The author and publisher shall in no event be held liable to any party for any direct, indirect, punitive, special, incidental or other consequential damages arising directly or indirectly from any use of this material, which is provided "as is", and without warranties.

As always, the advice of a competent legal, tax, accounting, medical or other professional should be sought. The author and publisher do not warrant the performance, effectiveness or applicability of any sites listed or linked to in this course.

All links are for information purposes only and are not warranted for content, accuracy or any other implied or explicit purpose.

Contents

What Is Acne?

Use Proper Cleansing To Treat Acne

Using Treatments To Fight Acne

Using Medications To Fight Acne

Prevention Is The Best Way To Treat Acne

Your Ultimate Guide For Acne Home Remedy

Acne Myths And The Perceptions They Cause

Acne Scars – Cause, Prevention And Treatment

Acne Skin Care Products

Dealing With Teen Acne

Acne Home Treatment 101

Products To Avoid When Treating Acne

Tips For Acne Prevention

Over The Counter Ideas For Treating Your Acne

Not All Scars Tell A Great Story

Misunderstanding Acne

Facing Acne: How To Cope With Its Effects

Acne Products Just For You

The Teenagers' Guide On Treating Acne

Effective Acne Treatment Options

What Is Acne?

New Treatments For Acne

Tips For Keeping Your Skin Acne Free

Acne Treatment: Do I Need to See A Doctor?

Acne Treatment: Exfoliating

Treating Acne With Topical Products

Treating Acne With Antibiotics

Treating Your Acne: Your Glands

Treating Your Acne With Natural Products

Preventing Acne From Happening

Acne - Not Just A Teenager's Nightmare!

LASER: Is This The Ultimate Cure For Acne?

Nlite Acne Scar Removal

Acne Treatments For Black Skin

Acne Treatment: What To Do When Acne Strikes

Adult Acne: The Three Main Sources

Treating Acne Using Tea Tree Oil

Cystic Acne - Causes And Treatment

How To Treat Back Acne

Laser Treatments To Help Cure Acne

The True Cause Of Acne

Understanding The Different Types Of Acne

Using Topical Products To Help Treat Acne

Ways To Treat And Prevent Acne Scarring

What You Should Know Before Taking Accutane

Acne Control The Natural Way: 8 Ways To Say Goodbye To Acne

Oral Acne Medication Options

3 Popular Myths About Acne

6 Acne Skin Care Tips

Coping With Adult Acne

How To Determine Your Skin Type

Natural Acne Treatment

Should You Use Makeup To Cover Up Your Acne?

Understanding Teen Acne

Understanding The Psychological Effects Of Acne

Water As A Natural Acne Remedy

What Causes Blackheads And How Are They Treated

When To Seek Medical Attention For Your Acne

What Is Acne?

Acne is a very painful experience for those that have to deal with it. For some individuals it will last only for a few years through their teenage years. For others, though, it will continue well into their future even until they reach 30 or 40 years of age. It is a skin condition in which bacteria or something else has irritated the skin and caused it to develop what are sores. These are red, pimple like masses that are not only uncomfortable, but can be damaging to the person's self esteem as well. Acne needs to be treated.

There are several things that can cause acne to happen on the skin. First, there needs to be right conditions for something to happen. The pores are often the place where it all happens. The skin is full of pores, tiny little openings on the skin. If these pores are full of oils that are secreted from your glands to keep the skin moist, then they are ideal places for bacteria to locate itself. If it is not washed away and killed, the bacteria will breed and soon they will be irritating your skin.

Acne can be treated in several ways. First of all, it should be treated by doing several of these things, as they are more likely to be beneficial when done together. First, the bacteria that is hitting and infecting the skin needs to be treated. For this to happen, the bacteria will need to be washed away. This can be done through exfoliating, through medicinal topical treatments or even with the help of lasers. The oil glands need to secrete only the right amounts of oil into the skin. This can be regulated by regulating the hormones that cause it. By taking care of these aspects, the individual's skin can improve, become healthier and eventually get rid of the infections that have been caused by the bacteria.

Use Proper Cleansing To Treat Acne

One of the first things that you can do to treat the acne that you have is to use the right types of cleansing products on it. There are several things that you can use and several ways in which you can use it to effectively stop the acne from getting worse as well as to help it to draw back and clear up. Taking care of your skin is the best way to treat the acne that you may have. It does not need to be that difficult to do either.

You can use a wide range of products to wash away the bacteria that hit your skin. If you look at them, make sure that you are not allergic to any of the products that are listed in the medication or cleansing product. Once this is seen, you can begin to see the results of use within a few weeks of use. The cleansers that you use should be that which is designed specifically for acne prevention and treatment. These will allow for the best results in the skin for your purpose.

You should also consider exfoliating. There are many products available that make this quite simple. The least harmful type is that of using pads or scrubs to do the exfoliation. All you need to do is to rub the product into the skin and it will remove dead skin cells from it effectively. You will also want to consider using moisturizers that are non oil based to help in keeping the skin hydrated. When you do this, you will have the best possible outcome for your skin. Proper cleansing of the face will provide you with the clean slate that you need that bacteria will not want to be in. The cleansers will be able to help you to get rid of the bacteria and the oil in your skin so that it can be free from the elements that cause acne.

Using Treatments To Fight Acne

There are many things that you will find available to you when it comes to treating your acne. There are many over the counter products that you can use to safely help you to get your skin back to where it used to be. When it comes to acne, no one likes it, but few know what they need to know in order to get rid of it. One of the things you will likely want to consider is that of the treatment programs that are offered throughout the web and throughout the drug store.

There are some benefits to using treatment programs. For one, you will have the best possible outcome to your acne treatment because many of these programs are all inclusive. That is, they provide for you all that your skin needs to get rid of the acne. When choosing them, though, you should learn a little more about them before you choose one over the other.

• What is the daily treatment plan? If this is something that is too challenging for you to do, then you are likely not going to stick to it and the program will then fail.
• The product should provide for a cleansing agent to help get rid of the oils in your skin, a moisturizer, especially if you are prone to dry skin, and it should include exfoliating products too. This combination can be the best treatment out there for acne.
• To know if the product will work for you, you will need to try it. Just because it worked for someone else does not mean you will have the same results. But, it can be a good idea for you to actually learn about how well it worked from others. What they did and did not like about it may be helpful in making a choice.

Using acne treatment programs can be a great way to get an all around benefit to your skin. If you do what the program says as much as you can, then you will have a good chance at seeing some relief from your acne.

<u>Using Medications To Fight Acne</u>

There are several different types of medications that can help you to get the best treatment out there for your acne. If you have acne and have tried using a wide range of cleansing products to help get rid of it, you may be frustrated with the fact that it has not cleared up. There are many treatment programs that are designed to help those that have moderate to severe acne, though. Even still, these too may fail to help you. Because each and every person needs something different, it is also necessary to call on your doctor for acne help through medications.

There are two types of medications that will generally be used. One is an antibiotic. The job of the antibiotic is to kill the bacteria that are the main culprit behind the acne. There are several medications that can be used in this manner. They can be used as topical treatments especially when the acne is confined to one or just a few small amounts of area. There are also oral antibiotics that can be used as well. These are ideal for those that are experiencing acne in larger areas of the body.

The second type of medication that is can be used is a hormone treatment. The glands that are under your skin are usually producing high amounts of oil. When you have acne, the bacteria will be attracted to these areas for the warmth and moisture. While antibiotics can treat the bacteria, the hormone treatments can work to stop or slow down the flow of oils. Most who have high levels of acne will have hormones that are all out of whack. Once they get this under control, the glands will go back to producing normal amounts of oil again.

Your doctor can help you to get the best answers to your questions about what is right and what will work for you. For some individuals, seeking out the help of your doctor can be the best course of action to take. It is often necessary, in fact, when individuals have severe acne.

Prevention Is The Best Way To Treat Acne

There are many medications on the market to help with acne. Some of these will work well for those that have acne. Some will not work for you. The best way to not have acne is to work on preventing it from happening instead of just waiting for it to happen and then treating it. This is the best way to go when you would like to keep your acne free or low acne infected face that way.

Tips

- *Use a good quality facial cleansing product.* These are available over the counter. If you know that you are likely to be one to get acne, then use those treatment programs that are designed for acne. You will find that there are many out there but choose the one that allows for the best fit to your specific needs. Use it twice per day, morning and evening.
- *Exfoliate your skin.* There are exfoliating products available to you as well. You should use them, as directed, to help you to get the dead skin cells off of your face as well as help you to get rid of the bacteria on your skin. If your skin becomes too dry when using these products, purchase and use a non oily moisturizer to help.
- *Eat a balanced diet that is full of the nutrients your body needs.* This will include lots of fruits and vegetables. Although this will not help with getting rid of acne, it will help your body to have a fighting chance at having what it needs to fight off infections.
- *Use a multivitamin.* If you are prone to acne outbreaks, you may want to consider a regiment that is designed for acne itself. These are ideal because they can provide for you a wide range of nutrients that most individuals do not get enough of.

Preventing acne means being proactive when it comes to it. If you would like to have the best results for your skin, then you should do whatever is necessary to secure this through prevention.

Your Ultimate Guide For Acne Home Remedy

Acne is an extremely common skin problem, occurring quite frequently amongst older teenagers and young adults. If ignored, acne can cause serious skin problems immediately or later in life. With all the different products out there to treat acne, you may be tempted to try some. But before you go out and purchase some of these often expensive products, try out some of these acne home remedies.

Toothpaste - For Minty Fresh Skin

Believe it or not, toothpaste can sometimes help clear up acne. While there have been no formal studies to date, many people swear by toothpaste as an effective acne home remedy. Simply apply directly to your problems spots before bedtime. Common wisdom holds that this will help control the swelling and redness. Just make certain you use actual toothpaste, not the gel stuff.

Salt and Vinegar - Pickle Those Zits

A solution of salt water, with or without vinegar, can help clear up your acne both by drying your skin (removing excess oils) and by helping disinfect. Wash your face twice a day with a salt water (and vinegar if you like) solution. Just don't make the remedy too strong, mildly salty is best. For stubborn spots, make a stronger solution, apply to the swollen area, and leave on for 15-20 minutes.

Fruits - Healthy Inside and Out

Fruits are also held to be an effective acne home remedy. Try applying strawberry leaves directly to the zit and leave the on for a while. Fresh lemon juice (not concentrated) or lime mixed with rose water is another acne home remedy you can try. Apply to your face and leave for 15 minutes. Try this one for 15 days and you just might be amazed at the results! Ground orange peel, mixed with water into a paste, can be effective in treating an outbreak. Apply and leave for 15-20 minutes, then rinse the paste off with warm water. Papaya juice is also widely held to be effective. Fresh tomato paste can be used much like the orange peel paste as well.

How To Win Your War Against Acne

The one thing all these fruit-based acne home remedies have in common is their astringent properties. Removal of excess oil and dirt is the key to fighting acne.

More Plant-Based Acne Home Remedies

In the same vein as the fruits discussed above, there are many herbs and plants that have also proven to be effective acne home remedies. A mixture of the oil extract of witch hazel, sweet fennel, and tea in water applied 2-3 times per day has been shown to be effective in fighting acne. Methi (fenugreek) leaves, crushed into a paste, can be useful when applied for 10-15 minutes before rinsing. Crushed garlic works as an effective acne home remedy as well, although most people forgo this one simply because of the smell. Aloe Vera has well-documented skin healing properties, and acts as an astringent as well. Cucumber, of course, has been a favorite to reduce all kinds of swellings for years. It can be more effective if you apply the cucumber in paste form. But I'll bet you didn't know that ground radish or ground sesame seeds are also another acne home remedy.

Support From the Inside

All these mixtures, concoctions, and pastes are nice to apply to the outside, but boosting your body from the inside makes any of these acne home remedies work that much better. Nettle tea has long been recommended as a cure-all for skin problems of all sorts, including acne. Taking a vitamin supplement with vitamin B5 and zinc promote a healthy immune system, helping your body fight off acne-causing bacteria. Give some of these home acne remedies a shot, and you just might be surprised at the results you can achieve without spending a ton of money on specialized skin care products.

Acne Myths And The Perceptions They Cause

Understanding what causes acne in the first place is an important step towards curing it. But it is easy to get caught up in the acne myths and avoid things that really have no relationship with your acne. Here are some of the more commons acne myths.

Acne Myth #1 - A Tan is Good for Your Acne

It is commonly myth that getting a tan can clear up your skin. Although it will cover up the redness, getting a tan does not help your acne clear up at all. In fact, the skin damage that can be caused by over-tanning can actually make your acne worse or complicate the healing process, as well as lead to more serious skin problems down the road.

Acne Myth #2 - French Fries Give You Acne

Since acne is caused by excess oils in your skin, it only makes sense that eating greasy foods or eating chocolate can cause acne, right? This is absolutely a myth. It has been scientifically proven many times that what you eat has no connection to your acne breakouts. So don't stop eating your favorite foods just because of an acne outbreak. It really doesn't effect your skin either way.

Acne Myth #3 - Washing a Lot Helps

While washing your face is an important part of controlling any acne, over-washing your face can strip your skin of essential oils and moisture. This will cause your skin to become irritated and dry, leaving it more susceptible to the infections that cause acne. The irritation will also slow the healing process of any existing acne. Washing is important, just don't overdo it!

Acne Myth #4 - Popping Your Pimples Clears Them Up

Again, while it may make sense to "clear out" the bacteria by popping a pimple, in reality this practice will push the bacteria deeper into the skin and leave open wounds where the pimple was. This can lead to secondary infections and scars, while furthering the spread of acne-causing bacteria at the same time. Devices that are made to help pop pimples or extract blackheads run the same risks of scarring. Don't pop those pimples!

Acne Myth #5 - Don't Wear Makeup

A lot of people say that wearing makeup causes acne. Yet again, this seems to make sense on the surface, since clogged pores lead to acne and makeup can get in your pores. But modern cosmetics often contain benzoyl peroxide or salicylic acid, which actually help fight acne.

There are many other acne myths out there. Understanding what causes acne and what not to do are important steps in treating your acne. If in doubt, or in severe cases, talk to your dermatologist about possible acne causes and treatments.

Acne Scars – Cause, Prevention And Treatment

Acne scars are easily recognized by the red skin of an area formerly occupied by a pimple. The initial form, while not actually a scar, will lead to one in some cases. Unfortunately, the only way to know for sure that it is a scar is if the red skin persists for longer than 6-12 months. It is often better, therefore, to treat all acne lesions as potential scars.

What Causes Acne Scars?

Acne scars are caused by an overabundance of the connective tissues your body uses to heal itself. These tissues work to provide a temporary framework for your skin cells to regrow on. But if there is too much of this connective tissue, it is not broken down when the healing is complete, but rather stays permanently. This causes a discolored or unpigmented section of skin to form.

Avoiding Acne Scars

Since the root cause of acne scarring is acne, preventing acne in the first place is the best way to avoid scars. But even if you already have acne, it is still possible to prevent acne scars from forming. The way this is done is by speeding the healing process as much as possible. The faster your acne lesion heals, the less time the connective tissue framework has to overgrow and leave scars.

Speeding the Healing Process

There are 2 main treatments dermatologists use to facilitate the rapid healing of acne lesions. The first is Tretinoin, an acid derivative of Vitamin A, also known as all-trans retinoic acid. This chemical speeds the skin's healing, reducing inflammation and preventing acne scars from forming.

The second method involves the use of various Alpha- and Beta-Hydroxy acids, which perform much the same function as Tretoinin, speeding healing and reducing the chance of scarring.

How To Win Your War Against Acne

Helping Yourself

Even if you don't or can't see a dermatologist, there are several different things you can do yourself that can help prevent acne scars from forming. The biggest thing is to treat your skin well. Avoid over-exposure to the sun, as sunburns can dramatically slow the healing process. Always wear sunscreen when going out in the sun. Don't pop your pimples, and if there are scabs from lesions, do not pick at them. Picking at any wound as it heals causes more damage, extending healing times and increasing the likelihood of scar tissue forming.

Removing Existing Acne Scars

Even with the best of care, scarring still sometimes occurs. But even if a scar does form, there are several options available that can reduce or eliminate your visible scarring.

Dermal Fillers

Fillers such as collagen can be injected into the site of an acne scar, raising the skin surface to reduce the appearance of pockmarks. These are not permanent treatments, however, and will require re-injection every 3-6 months.

Laser Resurfacing

An extremely popular and fast treatment for acne scars, laser resurfacing works by burning a precisely measured upper layer of skin. New skin then grows over the wound, leaving mostly unscarred skin visible. But as with the initial acne healing process, care must be taken to insure that this new skin does not scar as well.

Punch Excision

This procedure is only effective on certain types of scars. A surgical punch is made to precisely the dimensions of the scar to be removed. The scar is then punched out, similar to a cookie cutter, and the wound sewn together. If there is any scarring left after the wound heals, it can be more easily treated with laser resurfacing than the original larger scar.

Acne Skin Care Products

Keeping your skin healthy and acne-free takes some time, effort, and of course the proper acne skin care products. However, nearly everyone gets a pimple at some point in their lives. While teenagers are of course more prone to acne than adults, all age groups can benefit from proper use of acne skin care products.

Things to Keep in Mind

The biggest thing to keep in mind when shopping around for acne skin care products right for you is that everyone's skin reacts differently to various products. There are many different kinds of acne skin care products to choose from with widely different ingredients and formulas. If you have acne prone skin, your skin will probably tend to me more sensitive to the various chemicals you may wind up using. You should take it easy when trying out various acne skin care products. Check for a bad reaction before you cover your entire face.

Remember, what works for others may not work for you. The only way to find out for sure if it will work for you is to try an acne skin care product and see for yourself.

Facial Cleansers

Probably the most often-used acne skin care products are various facial cleansers. Try and find one that is gentle to your skin, and matched to your skin type. Oily skin needs different care than dry skin, for example. It is important to use a different kind of soap for your face than your body; most body soaps tend to be too harsh for use on your face, especially if you have active acne. But whatever you choose to use, stay with it. Changing to different chemicals or formulas, especially after using one specific brand of acne skin care product for a while, can cause more harm than good. And be careful of skin toners! They can dry your skin out, making you more prone to acne. If you use a toner, you should also consider using a moisturizer.

Moisturizers

If you are using any acne skin care products with benzoyl peroxide, you should consider using a moisturizer, since it tends to dry your skin. Most wipes and some facial cleansers contain

ingredients such as salicylic acid that can also dry your skin, so you should use a moisturizer as well.

Razors

Regardless of whether you use a bladed razor or an electric of some type, you must be very careful to avoid damaging your skin, especially if you have active acne. Keep the blades clean, and avoid cutting any blemishes you may have. The bacteria that cause acne can easily infect any razor nicks. The use of shaving cream can help prevent further irritating the skin. Whichever type of razor you use, you must be careful to avoid spreading or worsening your skin condition.

Healthy Inside, Healthy Out

Since acne is a bacterial infection, anything that boosts the body's ability to fight off infection can help keep you acne free and reduce the healing time of any acne you may have already. Taking a good multivitamin rich in vitamins a and c help your immune system, while vitamins B6 and E, for example, are good for your skin. Foods with lots of sulfur such as garlic and onions can help speed the recovery time of any acne you may have.

Final Thoughts

With such a bewildering array of acne skin care products out there, it may save you time and effort to go see a dermatologist. They can make recommendations based on their experience and point you towards the products that are right for you. They can also give you advice on proper use of any products they may recommend.

Dealing With Teen Acne

Acne is a major problem for those who have it. Not only are there major physical changes, but psychological changes as well. Formerly confident teens may find their self-confidence shaken by the way they look now.

Social Problems

Normal everyday social situations often become awkward and difficult for a teen suffering from acne to face. They will often try to avoid these social situations as much as possible. The teen may feel self-conscious and cut off from the group. There is a stigma associated with acne, and amongst teens especially, it is often considered to be a sign that a person is "dirty" or doesn't take care of themselves. All of this can make even going to class a painful experience for a teen. It erodes the teen's self-confidence, and sometimes these feeling will follow the teen into adulthood and cause depression and social maladjustment.

A Lack of Understanding

Many people who are not suffering from acne just don't seem to understand what the teen may be going through. They may think that the teen is just overreacting, and that it's "not that bad". But in recent years, the social and psychological side effect has been studied more closely. They found that acne is as much about how you think you look and how you feel emotionally, as it is the actual physical appearance. A teen's self-image and self-confidence can be fragile things while they are growing up, and having acne can cause the teen to have to deal with all sorts of unwelcome pressures and prejudices.

Modern society places a lot of emphasis in appearances, and anything outside the norm brings pressure to bear on the person breaking the "norm". When asked how they felt during these studies, teens with acne often said that they felt "ugly" and "depressed". These feeling can persist into adulthood, and are not gender specific. Both males and females felt similarly about their acne and how it made them feel.

Understanding What's Happening

How To Win Your War Against Acne

Understanding what pressures and feelings having acne can place upon your teen is very important, especially during the earlier teenage years. You must understand that acne is a big deal, and can leave lasting scars emotionally as well as physically. If you notice a change in your teen's behaviors, such as suddenly losing interest in social occasions, drop in grades, moodiness, etc., ask them what is bothering them. If it turns out that it is acne, don't just shrug it off. Take them to see a dermatologist, especially in the more severe cases. Make sure they understand that nothing they did is the cause of their acne, and that it will get better if they take care of it properly. Then make sure that they do take care of it properly.

Acne Home Treatment 101

Acne is a truly serious worry for teenagers and younger adults across the country. It can be a serious impediment to enjoying life while growing up. Mostly this is due to the undue importance our society places on appearances and being "normal" looking. In this article, we will examine several home treatments for acne in search of ways to clear your skin without emptying your wallet. Remember, clearing your skin can take time. Don't be discouraged if you don't see instant results when trying any of these home treatments.

Doing it Yourself

Treating your acne doesn't necessarily involve buying a bunch of expensive prescriptions or even over-the-counter products. All natural treatments can be made from common materials or plants that you probably already have around your house. The old favorite is toothpaste applied directly to the affected area. Simply apply the toothpaste to your zit before bed, and let it stay on overnight. Just make sure that the toothpaste you are using as a home acne treatment is actually the paste type, not the gel kind. You can also try a variety of solutions, pastes, and facial masks made from different plants, fruits, or vegetables. A simple salt and vinegar solution (be careful not to make it too strong) can be applied a few times a day to help dry out excess skin oils. Lemon, lime, or tomato juice can be used in a similar fashion. Herbs and herbal products (such as dried basil, mint juice, turmeric, and nutmeg) can be made into a solution or paste and used as well. Oatmeal masks are always popular, and cucumbers have been used to reduce inflammation for years. Some of the more exotic home treatments for acne are made from such ingredients as sandalwood, ground sesame seeds, papaya, ground orange peel, or fenugreek leaves. As you can see, natural home treatments for acne can be found in abundance.

The solutions, such as salt and vinegar solution, should be applied 2-3 times per day, with or without rinsing after 15 minutes. The pastes and other masks should be left on for 15 minutes, then rinsed away, and applied no more than twice a day. The honey and cinnamon mixture should be left on overnight if you are using this home treatment for acne. Remember, overdoing things can cause more harm than good. Give your skin time to heal, not more treatments. Most of the time you will notice a gradual decrease in the oil and pimples that are visible, with 15 days being the average time to notice a significant improvement.

How To Win Your War Against Acne

Over the Counter Treatments for Acne

If making pastes and extracts just isn't your thing, there are tons of over-the-counter treatments for acne. Benzoyl peroxide is one of the most common ingredients in commercial home treatments for acne. It helps remove excess oils from your skin, which is the main cause of acne. A good facial cleanser is important as well; you want a cleanser that will clean your face without over-drying, with just enough moisturizer to ensure that your skin stays smooth and soft.

Some Dos and Don'ts

Even with proper skin care, you will probably get a pimple at some point. When this happens, follow these tips to speed healing and minimize scarring.

DO keep the affected area clean.

DO continue to use your home treatment for acne.

DO use topical antibiotics (but not harsh ones like rubbing alcohol), especially if the lesion is raw.

DON'T pop a pimple.

DON'T squeeze blackheads.

DON'T pick at healing acne lesions.

<u>Products To Avoid When Treating Acne</u>

\With so many over-the-counter acne products available, how do you go about picking and choosing the ones that will work for you? There is no simple answer to this question, unfortunately. But there are things you can look for in a product, and certain things that you can avoid.

So which acne products are useful or helpful, and which kinds can aggravate your skin or cause damage? Let's look at some of the more common products used in acne treatment and prevention.

Soap

The first, and most common acne fighting product is good old-fashioned soap. Of course, there are many more choices nowadays than in our grandparent's day; unfortunately not all of the extras in soaps are good for skin trying to fight off or prevent acne. For one thing, the soap you wash your body with is probably way too strong for use on your face. Facial cleansers are the answer to this problem. They are specially formulated for use on the more delicate skin of your face. They can be had in forms made for all types of skin, from oily to dry or sensitive. Cleansers made for acne prevention or healing are generally oil-free, to avoid clogging your pores, have gentle cleansing agents, and an acne-fighting ingredient like benzoyl peroxide. And guys, if you don't want to be seen buying cream cleansers for your face, at least get a gentle, oil-free bar soap that rinses away easily for use on your face.

No matter which cleanser you wind up getting, don't overdo it. Wash in accordance with the directions on the product, and no more than once or twice a day in any case. Be gentle when washing as well. Scrubbing too hard can leave open wounds and cracks in your skin that acne bacteria can more easily invade. And don't pop you pimples! This can't be stressed enough. Popping your pimples forced the bacteria deeper into your skin and bloodstream, allowing them to spread, as well as greatly increasing the probability of scarring.

How To Win Your War Against Acne

Cosmetic

The wrong cosmetic can clog your pores, irritate your skin, and bring on an acne breakout. Fortunately, there are cosmetics available that are not oily, won't clog your pores, and even sometimes contain acne-fighting ingredients. No matter what, if a product causes skin irritation, stop using it and try a different product.

Choosing Acne and Skin Safe Products

Pay attention while shopping, and read the manufacturer's labels. These will often tell you what skin types the product is for, as well as ingredients and instructions. If you have oily skin, don't buy a moisturizing cleanser, for example. You need something that will help rid your skin of excess oils. People with dry skin, on the other hand, would use that product. If you have normal skin, you can probably use most products without too much trouble. But in all cases, test the products on a small, inconspicuous area overnight first, and check for irritation. If there is any, do not use that product. Unfortunately, there is no easy answer as to what acne product to choose. Everyone's skin is different, and what works for one person may cause you to get a rash (or just not help, more likely). Just try and restrict your choices to an intelligent subset based on your skin type, and you will find one that works for you.

Tips For Acne Prevention

Acne is a common topic of worry shared by teenagers the world over. Getting a zit at the wrong moment can feel like the end of the world, and since acne is more likely to appear during periods of stress, odds are that is exactly when you will see that pimple.

So What can you do about it? Well, there are many treatments out there that can help if you already have an acne breakout, both prescription and over-the-counter. But the best way to deal with acne is to try and avoid getting those pimples in the first place.

Keep Your Face Clean

Keeping your face (and the rest of you) clean is perhaps the single most important thing you can do to prevent acne. Getting rid of the dirt, excess oils, and bacteria on your skin is essential to preventing the acne before it starts. But don't over-wash; this can strip too much oil out of your skin, leaving it dry and vulnerable to infection by acne-causing bacteria. And if you already have acne, over washing will further irritate your skin, which could well make your condition worse.

You should probably get a special soap or acne cleanser for your face. The soap that you wash your body with is probably overly harsh for use on your face. The facial skin is much more delicate and vulnerable to harsh chemicals (including scents) and antibacterial. Acne cleansers are generally gentle and contain acne fighting ingredients to help prevent a breakout without irritating your skin or over-drying.

Keep it Cool

As we said above, stress is a major aggravating factor for acne. Try not to stress out too much (we know, easier said than done), and make sure you make time to relax every day. Get plenty of sleep, and make sure you eat properly. Taking a daily multivitamin can't hurt, either. Most people are lacking in some vitamin or the other, and a multivitamin can make up for any shortfalls in the days vitamin intake. Remember, vitamins are supplements, not replacements for regular meals. Staying out of stressful situations is a good idea, but let's face it, most stressful situations are ones we can't avoid. Just try and avoid the ones that you can.

How To Win Your War Against Acne

Dump That Skintight Shirt

If you are getting acne on parts of your body such as your chest or your back, wearing loose clothing for a while would be a good idea. Tight clothing abrades the delicate healing skin of a pimple, and can further spread acne-causing bacteria around the affected area. Loose clothing goes double for physically active activities, like working out or sports. Sweat will add to the irritating effects of tight clothing, and can increase your chances of a breakout if you don't currently have acne.

Don't Pop That Zit

Unfortunately, there is no 100% surefire way to prevent or heal acne. Sometimes, despite your best efforts, you will get the dreaded zit. Just take care of it as best you can, and do not pop it! You will be very tempted, and it seems like logically it could only help. But popping the zit causes further damage to the skin, and forces bacteria into the freshly created damage, spreading the acne further. Popping the zit also greatly increases the chance of scarring.

Over The Counter Ideas For Treating Your Acne

Pharmacies have numerous products designed to specifically treat all types of acne. Some products are created specifically to identify and address a specific purpose such as whitening the scaring, while others have been created with more general symptoms in mind.

This article will discusses a number of the more basic products presently being retailed over-the-counter which can help to prevent and address the symptoms of acne. Remember however that if products purchased over the counter aren't helping your skin condition, then it is advisable to seek professional medical attention.

As simple as it sounds, soap and water used appropriately is the most simple but one of the most effective products to help you to fight against acne. Depending on skin type, your sensitivity, and any allergies, you may choose a specific type of soap which will prevent additional breakouts or irritation for your skin type.

Washing your skin removes excess oils that may build up on all areas of your skin. It can help to un-clog the pores which cause pimples to form. Remember though that washing your face too often can cause as many problems as not washing enough. You should not scrub too vigorously or use too stringent a soap as that can remove too much oil and also irritate the skin further. Washing your face two or three times a day can help to remove unwanted oils and help control your breakouts without overdoing it.

Benzoyl peroxide is yet another common remedy which can be purchased cheaply and easily over-the-counter. It is effective at helping to fight acne. While it is quite often recommended by a range of physicians, it is often used to treat less serious forms of acne. Benzoyl Peroxide has been found to be helpful in fighting against bacteria. It stops excess oil build-up from clogging pores and is available in many forms including lotions or as a cream.

Another common treatment is salicylic acid. It is commonly used and forms part of a lot of over-the-counter cleansers and treatments. With milder occasions of acne, it can help to unclog blocked pores and prevent pimples but it does not prevent oil production. Similar to Benzoyl Peroxide, it needs to be used often in order to see the effects.

How To Win Your War Against Acne

Sulfur is another common product in numerous treatments. For years it has been used together with other products in an attempt to combat acne. Due to the unpleasant odor, sulfur is less often used by itself to treat acne.

Herbal and other natural products are available extensively for purchase quite often over-the-counter. Many are extremely effective to treat acne although other organic compounds have not been clinically tested to determine their effectiveness.

There are numerous over-the-counter treatments available to help heal or prevent acne. Different products will react differently to certain skin types so the effects are different on different people. It is important to determine what works well for you and then stick to it.

Not All Scars Tell A Great Story

Acne is not only about the spots and scars which mar your body. It is such a problematic ailment because it is not only the redness and irritation that causes you problems. Acne can lead to psychological and emotional stress which is much more dangerous than the physical problems. When thinking of treatments you need to think about both of these factors.

So just how widespread is acne?

If you look at the statistics, acne is one of the most common of complaints for all western countries. For Americans, forty to fifty million people face this problem daily. Most of them are teenagers or adolescents from the age of eleven up to young adults up to 30. Most commonly, they have poor skin across the face, neck, back and chest.

Choosing the correct type of treatment which matches your symptoms - the severity of the acne as well as where it is located - is important. Not all treatments would be appropriate for all people. To choose the correct type of treatment you need to have information to hand to assist you in your decision.

If your acne and physical appearance are bothering you then you have a range of things that you could use to address the problems, ranging from fairly mild to very invasive. You may want to try one or more of the following;

1. Autologous fat transfer
2. Collagen injection
3. Microdermabrasion
4. Dermabrasion
5. Skin grafting
6. Laser Treatment
7. Treatment of keloids
8. Skin Surgery

How To Win Your War Against Acne

All of the above treatments are available to you providing you have the agreement of a professional dermatologist. You may expect that only those with very significant scaring or facial disfigurement would be able to have the above treatments, but this is not the case.

The right way to treat acne scars must be determined well so that you are able to have the results you want and to make sure that you gat value for money.

Misunderstanding Acne

Once your acne starts to appear you may look for reasons for it, picking on excuses which are unreasonable and unrelated to what is really causing it. What is important is to look for the legitimate reasons why this may be happening rather than looking for excuses. It is also important to look for a cure rather than focus solely on the reason why you have it.

Here are some common reasons which people may focus on for causing acne;

Often, there is a misconception that Acne is unavoidable. People expect teenagers to develop it and link it to puberty of adolescence. While a change in hormones may be one contributing factor it is not inevitable or unavoidable. It is also not limited only to teenagers. Many adults develop acne at all stages of their lives, and hormone imbalance can be a contributing factor there also. Age does not matter as much as other factors. Cleanliness ,diet, open pores and being fastidious about hygiene is more important.

Stress is also believed by many to be a significant contributor to the development and continuation of acne. The media has even latched onto this as a reason and put forward the reduction of stress in your life as a possible way of reducing acne scarring. Again however, most scientific research agrees that this is a misconception. There is little evidence that there is a direct connection between stress and acne. Instead, things we have already mentioned such as personal hygiene, the way you live your life and healthy eating are more important.

When most individuals think of acne they treat it only as a physical problem. It is so much more than that. It is an emotional burden as much as a physical one. The psychological and emotional impact that acne causes can be more damaging than the physical ones. It can lead to a loss of self respect, low self-esteem and massive insecurity. It is the nature of the world in which we live that people focus on the outwardly physical rather than the kind of person we are. Those who have acne can become timid and insecure believing that others will label them 'ugly'.

But another, possibly one of the most common misconceptions is that acne can be picked up from oily foods, or eating too many sweets, desserts and poor food. it is true that a poor diet can contribute to it, but this is not the main reason. Do not give in to miss information or misconceptions. Be aware of what really does cause acne, and react accordingly.

How To Win Your War Against Acne

Facing Acne: How To Cope With Its Effects

Emotionally, acne can cause widespread effects to all age group but particularly adolescents. It is often the emotional or psychological effects rather than the red spots or disfigured skin which leave the greatest scars. Creams and potions, face peels and masks can be excellent physical cures, but learning to live with yourself can be the hard part.

Since acne is so common in teenage years, the social insecurity amongst teenagers is significant in shaping social activity. For teenagers living through the trauma of acne, it is often difficult to accept the social impacts that acne brings. Spots can be seen as marks of shame, cause depression and even lead to self-pity. Parent of teenagers who face this problem are integral to providing the help a person needs. So as a parent, what can you do?

You can remind your children that acne is a temporary condition - As a guardian or a parent you should be aware of what is happening and give encouragement. You may see them unhappy because of the way in which people criticize or tease. Remember to tell them that acne and poor skin conditioning will not last long and that in time the condition will be cleared up. Continue to explain how important it is to move on and ignore comments despite any negative reaction from other people. Words are not important over time.

Take your teenager to a dermatologist - You should never wait for your teenager's acne to develop into a problem or get worse. Be proactive and take him or her to see a dermatologist. It is important to do this earlier rather than later. And, you need to use a dermatologist who engenders your trust. Go to see them with your child as they progress through their treatment with their dermatologist.

Guide your teenager or child to be responsible - There are some activities that may make acne worse. Make sure that you are close enough physically and spiritually to be in a position to remind them of their responsibilities. Explain the reasons behind acne and be sure to answer any questions that your teenager has.

Boost your teenager's self-image - Self-confidence plunges when others mock and tease. The effect on any teenager can be bitter, so as a parent or guardian you really need to be there to counteract the loss of self-esteem he or she faces. Be generous with your praises but do not

spoil your child. Tell your teen about how wonderful his or her talent is. This would be a lift to his/her morale.

You are a parent, and you can help your teenager to feel better about themselves even as a person with acne. Remind them that this is just a stage; it will surely come to an end. Be there and support your child like no one else can.

Acne Products Just For You

Acne, a universal problem for all kinds of people of all ages has resulted in a plethora of Acne products flooding the market. They come at a range of prices, packaging and strengths but they have a common aim - to eradicate pesky pimples that make your life a misery. Here, we outline a few of them for your choice;

Acne Product One: Astara Blue Flame Purification Mask

This mask was created to be soothing and refreshing and to work in a short time span. A fifteen minute application will increase the healthiness of your skin, opening the pores and improving your appearance. As well as addressing acne that already exists it is also billed as preventing the future appearance of spots.

Acne Product Two: PhytoMe Acne Gel

This product is especially effective against all types of skin complaints including whiteheads and blackheads! The formula is designed specifically to be non-drying and is formulated to help your skin to relax. This specially advanced acne gel can address even the most entrenched pimples on your face. Use it regularly to help further breakouts of acne in the future.

Acne Product Three: Neutrogena Cooling Gel Masks

These masks are not intended to cure existing break outs of acne. They are designed to cool and rejuvenate the face, clean the skin and invigorate the pores. If they are used regularly they have a secondary knock-on effect in controlling the reoccurrence of acne. It is a refreshing experience and soothes the face and it does an excellent job of cleaning up the skin.

Acne Product Four: Acne Dry Spot

These products are designed to be applied before bed and to work through the night. Applied to any inflamed area before retiring for the night, it is effective at zapping those spots as you sleep. It is especially made to address existing zits so don't make the mistake of applying this to unaffected areas as a preventative measure. If you were to you might end up with damaged

skin. If you see a spot about to be emerge, apply a small amount of this and the acne spots will be stopped in their infancy.

Acne Product Five: Biore Blemish Bomb

As the name suggests this product is a powerful weapon when it comes to attacking skin problems. It can be used for as few as two days, and you can now zap problem spots into oblivion. It is applied as a liquid but then dries to form a protective covering over your acne. Once morning comes, peel away this protective patch and uncover a much reduced skin problem.

Acne Product Six: pHisoderm 4-Way Daily Acne Cleanser

Get more than your money's worth with this powerful acne product. This is the ideal four-in-one combined product which works as a toner, a cleanser and a spot fighter to boot! It will clear the problem area in a few short weeks when applied twice daily. As well as tackling existing spots it also helps to reduce the recurrence by unclogging your pores. It is compatible with all skin types and will prevent dryness and irritation.

Acne Product Seven: DDF BP Gel 5% using Tea Tree Oil

Here nature and medical research team up with this product to attack your acne. Highly effective, this product is designed to obliterate all spots in just a few days. It helps to fight new and emerging break outs. Drying of the skin may be felt initially but just following the instructions will avoid significant skin irritation and soreness.

Acne Product Eight: Derma Clear

This is another multi-use product to address acne. This acne-zapping wonder will not only address simple pimples but also cleanses and rejuvenates the skin if it is used daily.

The Teenagers' Guide On Treating Acne

Acne without doubt is one of the most widespread problems facing teenagers anywhere in the world. For some, acne can be a truly horrendous experience, while for others it can have little or no impact at all. But for those it does affect it can lower their self-esteem and limit their ability to express themselves openly and confidently. It can impact on friendships and even on family relationships.

I can leave emotional scars and cause embarrassment to such an extent that they may not even wish to leave their rooms!

But acne is a natural, normal occurrence. As such it should not be viewed with dismay and certainly should not be taken so seriously as to lead to depression. Recent statistics suggest that it effects 90% of teenagers at one time or another, and about a quarter of adults.

But as a natural occurrence acne can be treated. Doctors and health professionals nowadays are able to provide very powerful, effective acne treatments for all ages but particularly teenagers. It is well worth following tips and suggestions and following a decent health plan. Prevention is better than cure, and the best cure for acne is to be vigilant and take preventative measures. If however you already have acne there are some excellent ways to address it;

Self-prepared remedies

Many acne treatments for teenagers can actually be found very easily, most often from ingredients already available inside your home or garden. Fruits and herbs are known to provide cures for almost any health problem, and one of these is acne.

As well as achieving a cost effective, powerful treatment you may find it fun to create your own proven acne treatment which can be used by everyone including teenagers. Creating a paste to be used on one spot or as a mask is quite straightforward and an excellent idea.

The first type would be to make a mixture of ground orange peel or fresh lemon juice.

How To Win Your War Against Acne

Another effective acne treatment for teenagers is actually a mixture of tea tree and sweet fennel essential oils added with witch hazel. This is believed to remove the excess oil and dirt on your face and kill the bacteria that cause the unwanted acne. Corn flour mixed with egg white is another great option that you can try to clear that acne in your face. Cucumber, a favorite acne treatment for teenagers, is tested to prevent the appearance of acne. It also refreshes your tired and unhealthy skin.

Right on the counter

When you think home-made preparations are not the acne treatments for teenagers like you, then 'over-the-counter' products are more recommended for you. Anytime at the nearest store in your neighborhood, you can buy these non-prescription products that are truly great acne treatments for teenagers. Boys especially prefer these products for it is really awkward for them to put on a facial mask. Benzoyl peroxide is actually the best known acne treatment for teenagers that is available in stores. It works as to dry the skin and eventually encourage it to peel off and form a new, healthier skin surface. It also has antibacterial effects, very good in killing that irritable acne-causing bacteria.

The doctors' advice

Not all cases of acne problems can be treated by self-made applications or "over-the-counter" drugs. These actually only treats mild to moderate acne problems. Thus, a consultation with your doctor is advisable, especially when you have a severe case of acne problem. Your doctor will surely give you more potent acne treatments for teenagers which are actually divided between topical and oral solutions. Topical acne treatments given to teenagers are applied directly on the skin include antibiotic lotions and azelaic acid which is described as a benzoyl peroxide alternative. Meanwhile, oral antibiotics that you have to take in are just some of the recommended acne treatments for teenagers.

Effective Acne Treatment Options

Acne is one of the most common of skin disorders. It often starts in adolescence and mainly afflicts the teenage age group. With 70% of adolescents afflicted with this common skin problem, it is often considered to be one of the most irritating diseases especially during an adolescent's life. Although it may not always be serious in the sense that is not fatal, it can cause serious emotional trauma to any person ridiculed because of their complexion.

There are numerous medical interventions to help people of all ages to resolve their acne problems. Physicians and researchers are continually seeking the ultimate treatment and the question always is as to which is the most effective. Natural and artificial compounds are continually being tested and combined in an attempt to make a super-treatment.

Here is a breakdown of a number of acne treatments which claim to be successful in dealing with different types and severity of acne spots;

Mild and Juvenile Acne

This kind of acne - often described as teenage spots - can be effectively treated using over-the-counter (OTC) medicines available in most good drugstores. This kind of acne is considered to be amongst the easiest to treat but many prescription medical interventions are also effective as acne treatments. These include a range of antibiotics, adapalene, benzoyl peroxide and tretinoin. These treatments help prevent or stunt the development of bacteria and decrease inflammation and reddening.

Depending on the person's skin type a doctor may choose to prescribe an acne treatment they believe to be appropriate and effective. As an example, if a patient has oily skin then certain creams and lotions would not be advisable, mainly as these are oil-based medications. Certain Gels and liquid solutions will be more suitable in this case since they are predominantly alcohol-based and therefore tend to dry out the skin.

Physicians and medical researchers would test a vast range of treatments before allowing them to market, and individual physicians would test a number of products on their patients before committing to a specific course of treatment for any one person. Because there is such a range of options this is very prudent.

How To Win Your War Against Acne

Moderate or more severe acne

Those who have oily skin or those who used to have a form of mild acne (often this is in their later teens and early twenties) may experience worsening acne as they grow older. This may develop into a moderately severe form of acne requiring more advanced intervention. Moderately severe acne is often characterized by an increased number of whiteheads and increased redness around sores. This is often due to ruptured blood vessels.

Severe acne is categorized as when it has spread to cover a larger area, often the entire face, or parts of the back and neck. Often this will involve the development of larger spots and this type of acne is often treated with oral antibiotics. They work by preventing or reducing the development of bacteria which can contribute to or cause acne and reducing any inflammation. When dealing with this increased level of acne a combination of medications may be required. Often oral medication and skin rubs or creams used together may be necessary. Certain topical medications such as sulphur drug preparations have been considered extremely effective as acne treatments. Sulphur creates a peeling effect on your skin and this loosens the poor dead skin and can dislodge blackheads from their pores. Sulphur has no known side effects and as such is an effective acne treatment.

However it is always advisable to test any medication on a small area of your skin before applying them, and only take medicines oraly if instructed to do so. Examples of effective acne treatments come in the form of oral antibiotics are tetracycline, minocycline, isotretinoin, doxicycline and erythromycin.

Most of these effective acne treatments when taken orally are deemed hazardous to pregnant women and their children's health. Of the above, only erythromycin is reputed to be safe for use by those who are either expecting a baby or breastfeeding.

What Is Acne?

If you are one of the thousands that will purchase acne treatment products this year, before you invest your money, you need to know several things about what is happening to your face, your chest and your body. Often, individuals blame the acne on their body on puberty. But, it can be caused by many more things as well. For some, it is just this, puberty. For others there are other conditions that may be causing the acne to appear. If you take the time to understand why you have acne, you are likely to learn how you can treat your acne.

Acne is an infection on your skin. Normally, it happens because bacteria get into your pores where it breeds. Once the skin becomes irritated by this, it will then react in the form of sores. This is the acne that you see on your face.

Acne is generally caused by the occurrence of the bacteria on your face and increased amounts of oils on the face which make it a welcoming place for bacteria to go and hide. These two things are generally the case for most types of acne. But, there are different things that cause them to happen. This is what you need to learn in order to know how to treat your bacteria.

- The oils that are being secreted at high levels may be due to hormone imbalances that are caused by such things as puberty, stress, health issues and other conditions.
- Bacteria can get onto the face from a poor level of keeping your face and your skin properly cleaned.
- Bacteria can feed on the dead skin cells that are not properly exfoliated away, making this a more likely target for growth.
- Eating a poor diet can help to encourage oily skins as well as lowers the body's ability to fight off the infections that it is facing.

To learn what is causing your acne problems, you should carefully think about what is happening in your life and improve anything that you may see as an obvious reason why your body may be facing these factors. In most cases, you will need to seek out the help of your family doctor or a dermatologist when it comes to determining your body's reasons for over producing oil secretion in your skin. This can be done through a blood screening or in some cases your doctor may not need to do anything to realize that this problem needs to be addressed. These are the first steps in getting rid of your acne.

New Treatments For Acne

If you are looking for the most advanced techniques for treating acne, there are many to choose from. Usually, there are many things that contribute to acne. There are many over the counter products that you can use to treat your acne too. If you do not like them, or they do not seem to work well for you, you may decide to go off to see your family doctor or your dermatologist for help. He or she may recommend medications to control your hormone levels and to regulate the amount of oils in your glands or they may want you to take antibiotics that will kill off the bacteria. Yet, even this is not a fully fool proof way of fighting off acne.

If you are ready for some real world help there are many things that you can do. One of the first things that you can consider is that of lasers. Laser surgery, actually, can be a very beneficial method to treating acne. If you are like many, you are not looking for something that is a magic potion, but something that will work over time. That is what lasers can do. They will do several things. First, they are likely to destroy or damage the follicle that the hair is growing from. They will also destroy or damage the gland that is producing the excess oils that are in your skin. And, finally, they will also help in killing the bacteria that is causing the acne too.

Lasers are very effective and minimally invasive. There is little to no signs that you have had the procedure done either. While it is not going to be able to remove the acne that you already have, it can help it to lessen and then help to prevent more from resurfacing. The goal here is to find the solution for your needs that offers the best ability. If you believe that laser surgery is the way to go, then consider this option. You may need several treatments and they can be rather expensive, but they can be quite beneficial nonetheless.

Laser treatment for acne is something that is becoming more and more effective. Many people are using them not only to treat the acne that is on their face and the acne that is going to be there if they do nothing about it, but it can even help in hiding or getting rid of acne scars as well. Acne can be treated with lasers.

Tips For Keeping Your Skin Acne Free

There are many things that you can do in order to enable yourself to keep acne at bay. There is no fool proof method that will work for everyone when it comes to acne removal, but there are many things that may be able to help you to control it. You may be able to prevent it from happening to you. Or, you may be able to lessen the amount with which is happens. In any case, treating your acne is something that you will need to do, especially when you are facing severe cases of it.

Proper Cleansing

Because acne is mainly caused by bacteria that get into the pores on your face, the first real thing that you need to do is to keep this from happening. While there is no way to stop it from getting onto your face, it is possible for you to remove it before it becomes a problem. You should purchase a good quality cleansing product. There are many on the market but you will want to look for those that have antibacterial qualities to it. This will help to rid your skin of bacteria.

No matter how well you wash your face, though, there may still be bacteria lurking there. Another thing that you should do to help keep it at bay is to use exfoliating products. The dead skin cells that are on your skin can contribute to your level of acne. First, they can actually block your pores and contribute to the oil blockage which in turn can lead to acne. The dead cells also can be used by bacteria as a food source so that they can breed. Removing them is quite simple, though. You will simply need to use exfoliating skin care products which are readily available.

When That's Not Enough

For many individuals, just washing their face and skin properly is enough to lower the amount of acne that they face. For others, though, this is not enough. These individuals should seek out the help of their dermatologist. It may be necessary to use products to help regulate the oil production in the skin. Medications can help by turning off the oil glands there.

When it comes to treating and preventing acne, there are many products on the market that can help. The most effective thing that you can do, though, is to insure that you use them regularly as directed. Most of them need to be used on a regular basis if they are to help. Not everyone can have a clear complexion, but many will find relief in these products for acne prevention as well as acne treatment.

Acne Treatment: Do I Need to See A Doctor?

Many parents worry about their teenager's acne levels. Although acne is commonly found in many teens and even well past this stage, it is still something that can trigger a reaction from parents. Many of those that do experience acne should seek out the help of a doctor. Realizing that acne does not only scar the face and the other areas of the skin where it is found, but it also hurts the self esteem of those that have it. Many will feel embarrassed or will hate the way that they look. Seeking out the help of a doctor may be something that can be done. Before you do this, though, you may want to find out if you have done everything that you can to insure that this is the right step to take.

The first thing that needs to be done is that the individual needs to insure that proper cleansing of the face is done. Now, normally every day washing of the face can help, but is most of the time not enough to help prevent or treat acne. To make it more effective, the individual that is facing the acne should consider using products that are designed to pull out the oils and bacteria in the skin to help clear up acne. These products are designed to help the skin to heal too.

Many of these products will contain products such as peroxide or alcohol in them. This will help to dry out and remove the oils as well as help to kill off the bacteria causing the acne. Another product that may be important to use are those exfoliating products that can be purchased over the counter. These will work away the dead skin cells on the face and help to remove debris that is in the pores.

When these things are done, the next thing to look at is the diet and the stress levels of the individual. While the diet that you eat has little to do with how much oil your body produces, by eating a well balanced diet you will be allowing the body to have the nutrients that it needs to heel and fight off any infections that it may face. Stress can also trigger acne inadvertently. Here, the body will react with the over production of hormones including those that trigger oil production in the skin.

When all of these things are done and there is still a problem with acne, which may just be the case, then it may be time to call on your family doctor. This individual may be able to help or they may refer you to a specialist called a dermatologist. In any case, working with these individuals can help you to get the best results for your acne.

Acne Treatment: Exfoliating

There are many things that you can do to help to improve your skin's condition when it comes to acne treatment. One of them is exfoliation. This is the process of using a non harmful but slightly abrasive product to rub and wash against the skin. Like most other types of acne treatment, it is common for these products to help when worked in conjunction with others. Yet, exfoliating the skin can be one of the best ways to treat acne.

There are several different types of products that you can use for exfoliating. It can be done through a mechanical element such as an abrasive scrub product or a liquid soap which are made for the use of exfoliating. These are the most common types of products used for exfoliating. Exfoliating can also be done chemically by using products such as salicylic acid as well as glycolic acid. These products will help the skin to peel back the top layer of it. It is nothing that you will see happening and in most case you will not feel anything bad. The goal here is to use these products to help remove the top layers of the skin where dead skin cells are. These cells get into the skin through the pores and block them. This blockage along with the over production of oils that happens in the skin can encourage acne. These products can be used as both preventative measures or as a treatment for existing acne.

When you have acne that is already present on your skin, you can use exfoliating products that are designed as treatment products. You should take note though that you do not want to cause pain to your face especially in those sensitive acne areas. Always use the products as directed for the best results and the right reaction on your skin.

In some cases, exfoliation can cause visible flaking of the skin. This is generally normal and should not be anything to alarm you. You may want to purchase moisturizers for your skin that are not oil based to use after the exfoliating process. You may want to consider these because the skin can become quite dried out and irritated. You will find these moisturizers available with the exfoliating products. Look for those that can be used in conjunction with each other for the best results. Exfoliating is a good way to work on healing or preventing acne on your face and throughout the rest of your body. Always follow the manufacturer's directions, though, to insure the best possible outcome.

Treating Acne With Topical Products

If you walk into the acne treatment aisle at your local drug store, you are likely to find a wide range of products that are designed to help you. There are many that are creams, lotions, pads and all sorts of other products. Yet, one thing is for sure. You will be overwhelmed with which ones you should be choosing. Some that you may want to consider are the topical products for treating acne. There are many of these too, but understanding what they are and how they work will allow you to make the best choice for your acne. They can help to prevent acne too.

Most of the over the counter types of topical creams that you can use will have Benzyl peroxide in them. This is like a mild type of bleach product that is safe to use on your skin. The product needs to be used regularly and will help to prevent new acne formations from happening. You should always use them according to the directions that are provided by the manufacturer. Generally, they will be applied to the face or affected area twice per day. This is usually done once in the morning and once before bed. It is rubbed right into the skin so that it penetrates the pores. This will help you because it will kill P. Acnes, which is the type of bacteria that gets into your pores and created acne.

Using these products does have its advantages. Unlike using antibiotics, products with benzyl peroxide actually is stronger than them and does not allow for any resistance. When using these products, though, you may feel that your skin is becoming dry or even that there is added redness to it. You may experience irritation as well. To help this, you can often find non oil based moisturizers to help you.

Using these products is quite common. You can find a wide assortment available to you throughout your drug store shelves. When choosing which one to use, look for those that can work at your level of acne. For those that have mild or moderate levels, these can be quite beneficial in helping to slow or stop the acne. If you have sensitive skin or dry skin, there are specialty products that are available to you to use as well. In order for these products to work for you, though, you simply must use them on a regular basis as directed by the manufacturer.

Treating Acne With Antibiotics

Because acne is caused at least in part from bacteria, it is very helpful to many to actually use antibiotics to help treat the condition. There are several options that can work for you, depending on what is causing your acne and your doctor's decision on how to treat them. It is necessary for you to seek out a doctor to help in the purchase of prescription antibiotics, but many are given by family doctors for patients that are in need.

The antibiotics that can be used to treat acne can do so in the form of either a topical product or an oral antibiotic. It has been shown that they offer about the same type of help no matter how they are used and applied. Topical products can actually be better for some individuals because they do not cause any real side effects that ingesting can cause such as stomach problems and drug interactions with other medications that you are taking. The most common types of antibiotics for topical treatments of acne include clindamycin, erythromycin and in some cases tetracycline.

On the other hand, oral antibiotics can be beneficial as well as topical products. If you have a large area that is in need of treatment, these can be quite difficult to treat with topical ointments. It can be easier then to just take the medication orally. The oral options to treat acne include tetracycline or erythromycin. These are the most common options for oral antibiotics for acne treatment. These medications can help you to stop the bacteria that is irritating your skin and therefore causing it to be irritated, but this does not, by itself, improve the acne that you have. As soon as the bacterium gets to the pores, again, you still have a problem.

It is necessary to treat acne in several ways, in most people. Usually, it is the combination of factors and treatments that allows you to get the most benefit from acne relief. Antibiotics like these can and do help with the relief of acne but they do much better when they are combined with other methods. Often, the problem lies in how much oil the skin is absorbing. When this is the case, it is essential that the oil glands are regulated at well or you will just be attracting new bacteria to the pores. If you stop taking your antibiotics and still have the right opportunities for acne to reappear, it can be only a few weeks to even a few days until you see acne forming again.

Treating Your Acne: Your Glands

There are several things that go into making acne. Your skin needs to provide a warm area that is moist as well as has the ability to house the bacteria that cause acne. You will need the bacteria, which is only attracted to the skin when the conditions are right and there's a food supply. With that said, your skin is the likely target for many acne outbreaks because it is generally oily, full of dead skin cells that can be a source of food and it offer pores which are ideal places for bacteria to gather and breed. Let them find someplace else to hide because you can help to stop acne on your body.

One of the elements that contribute to acne is that of the oils that your skin is producing. During puberty, which is the highlight of the acne career on your body, the oil glands that are lurking under your skin are working over time to produce a high amount of oil. They are told to do this, though. The hormones that are in the body at this time are fluctuating and this causes the body to respond in strange ways. One of them is to produce more oil then is needed. The problem with this is that the oils are very attractive to the bacteria that are looking for a home in your skin.

You can do many things to treat the acne on your face and many of them will revolve around treating the actual bacteria that is causing the acne. But, for many, this is not enough to turn off the acne machine that your skin has become. You often need to turn off those oil glands so that it is not so inviting to live in your pores. To do this, there are several medications that your doctor can provide you with. Their goal is to control the hormones in your body.

By regulating the hormones that your body is experiencing, they can better get those oil glands under control. Some of the most commonly used treatments include oestrogen/progestogen contraceptive pills. Also, anti-testosterone Cyproterone used with oestrogen can actually be quite helpful in treating acne.

By understanding just what is causing the acne on your skin from happening you can be better aware of the things that you need to do in order to prevent it from getting worse and you can work to improve it. If your skin is over producing oils, then it may be helpful to you to seek out the help that your doctor can provide for you.

Treating Your Acne With Natural Products

Acne treatments are often something that many are searching for. Yet, many of the products that you will purchase that are over the counter products from your local pharmacy are those that are filled with chemicals and man made products. If you visit your doctor's office for help with your acne, you may find that here too, many of the medications that he can provide for you are chemicals as well. For those that do not like to fill their bodies with chemicals, there are natural remedies for treating acne that may just work well for you.

Natural remedies are things that are naturally occurring in the world without the help of a human. These products are ideal because they do not cause nearly the same high levels of reactions and side effects of that of chemical products. They also do not provide for as many reactions with the medications that you may already be taking. Finally, natural products are just simpler for your body to take and use in the best way possible.

What Options Are There?

There are many things that you can do to get natural products into your body to help you to fight acne. Many of these products are those that you would find normally in foods. The very best way to help yourself, in this case or any other, is just to naturally consume the right foods to aid your body in fighting bacteria, regulating itself and just to help it to stay healthy. Eating a well balanced diet, one that is rich in vitamins and minerals is the best action that you can take to start with.

Here are some types of supplements that may be able to help you in your battle against acne:

- **Zinc.** This product is a natural element that you need in your diet anyway. It has been shown to be quite effective at treating inflammatory acne. It may not be as beneficial as some of the medications, both oral and topical, that you can use, but it does help when trying to avoid these products.
- **Chromium:** This supplement has been shown to help in some cases as well.
- **Multi vitamins:** In many ways, a good multi vitamin can offer overall help to you too. You can even find combinations that are put together for the specific purpose of acne treatment.

Using natural methods to relieve your acne can be one of the most beneficial things that you can do simply because it is often the case that nature knows what is best for your body.

Preventing Acne From Happening

It almost seems like overnight there are acne problems for many teens. Yet, acne is not something that just happens overnight. In most cases, it happens over time any place from several weeks to several days. When you realize that there are things that you can do to prevent it, though, you may be more proactive in making sure that your skin's condition is in the best shape possible to avoid this happening to you. Many individuals will find themselves wondering what to do now that they have acne, but before you get it, you can do much to stop it from happening.

The skin is the prime location for bacteria to find a home. If you make sure that it is not a welcoming spot, your skin will appreciate it and you will not worry every time you look into the mirror. There are several things that you can do including the following.

- *Use antibacterial soaps when washing.* These can be the best bet when it comes to fighting off the bacteria that will find your pores at some point. Make sure to wash your face twice per day, in the morning and in the evening before bed. You may want to consider using acne medications to help you in prevention too. These are over the counter cleansing products that can help to wash away debris, kill off bacteria and keep up the excessive oils on your face.
- *Exfoliate.* Here too you can improve your skin's appearance long before it is hurt by acne by simply using exfoliating products. These will help you to strip the bacteria from the face and will also help in removing the dead skin cells that are blocking your pores. Over the counter products can help here too.
- *Exercise, eat right and stay stress free.* These things do play a role in your body's ability to fight against the bacteria hitting your skin. If you provide your body with what it needs to get rid of it faster, you will see better results all around.

Prevention is the best medicine when it comes to your face, your skin and acne. There are many such products on the market that can help you to do this. You can even find supplements that can help your body to ward off acne. With some help, you can prevent the worst types of acne from afflicting you.

Acne - Not Just A Teenager's Nightmare!

Though acne is associated with adolescence the fact is that it is more prevalent in adults than just teenagers. It has observed that a majority of teenagers who have suffered from attacks of acne are not easily affected by the malady. If you thought that acne was only for teenagers then prepare to be surprised when you actually discover the number of adults battling this ugly skin disorder all over the world.

The many physical, psychological and behavioral effects acne has on teenagers and adults alike are common allover the world and are the cause of a great many problems being faced by those people affected by this disorder. Recent research has disclosed that the disorder is on an upward swing in adults though the exact cause is not known as yet.

The physical and psychological effects of acne are long-lasting irrespective of when acne strikes its victim. Acne can strike in adolescence and last long enough to see one through to adulthood or for the more fortunate ones it might decide to just up and leave within a few weeks or months of discomforting the afflicted. Acne can also strike when the person is over 30 so beware, nip the disorder in the bud by consulting a dermatologist as early as possible.

Skin experts are of the opinion that when acne strikes in an adult the effects are very long lasting and can also leave permanent scars since the skin loses collagen due to aging, which finds it difficult to recuperate from the disorder and so has to contend with permanent scars caused by acne.

A common misconception with the more devastating psychological scarring caused by acne is that adults are better equipped to handle the disorder and so can handle the adverse social effects of acne than most of our teenagers are. In actuality the effects of these psychological scars are more severe than believed. Because acne is believed to be a disorder associated with teenagers and adolescence many adults find it difficult to admit that they are afflicted by acne. This makes it more difficult to manage in early stages where it can be effectively treated.

Times are changing for the better with more research proving that the many beliefs surrounding acne are more misconceptions than facts. This is allowing many people to seek timely help from medical practitioners and dermatologists including beauticians many of whom prescribe

How To Win Your War Against Acne

medication that are known to effectively treat acne in the early stages. There is a plethora of information available about acne and this is a great help in removing the many misconceptions about this disorder.

It is not like acne will last a lifetime. Acne will vanish ultimately even without treatment, though this may take a very long time. When one discovers the onset of acne they should seek timely help from a qualified dermatologist and follow the advice given to the 'T'. This will help in relieving acne earlier and without the many discomforts associated with the disorder.

LASER: Is This The Ultimate Cure For Acne?

Contrary to popular belief acne a skin disorder that afflicts both adults as well as teenagers. Acne is not very easily cured but skin specialists are armed with a newer technology that promises to get rid of this ugly skin disease permanently - Laser treatment!

Unlike past beliefs acne is a skin disorder that seems to be afflicting more adults than teenagers in modern times. Perhaps this was the case in the past too however it is only now that adults are acknowledging the fact that they have acne and are coming forward to deal with the problem at the very onset of the disorder. Though there are a variety of treatments for acne most of them are very time consuming and take a very long time to begin to show some results if any. From using prescription drugs to skin applications (not recommended) to turning to non-prescription medications over the counter people suffering from acne have tried them all mostly to their dismay when they realize that the acne is still very much there.

The cases where people have successfully treated acne by self medication are rare. Doctors prescribe very potent drugs that have also known to have failed. This is when they turn to technology and decide to try out laser treatment. It is believed that laser treatment, when carried out by a specialist, can completely cure acne permanently. But then there are cases where laser treatment has taken a very long time and the treatment is not complete. But where laser treatment has actually worked the results are astounding. Laser treatment for acne is a technology that has given many people suffering from this skin disorder a lot of hope and solace.

Laser treatment for acne scarring has been used successfully or many years with just a few people responding poorly to the treatment, but the number of poor responses are negligible. The big question people ask is whether laser treatment for acne is safe and effective for a long period of time. The answer to that query has been answered many times with the objective of trying to convince acne patients to turn to the treatment which is very effective.

So How Is This Treatment Administered?

The extreme heat produced by the laser apparatus damages the sebaceous glands. The heat is applied for a split second and so it does not burn the skin of the patient and very little or no

How To Win Your War Against Acne

discomfort is experienced by the patient. It is possible to use laser to treat acne at least four treatments with a thirty day break between each treatment session. A majority of the patients undergoing laser acne treatment are 100% rid of the disorder. The sebaceous glands are altered by the extreme heat from the laser device and fail to produce oil, this is immediate evidence that laser treatment is an effective acne cure.

There are two laser technologies that are used to cure acne. One technique attacks the bacteria growing in the glands causing acne and the other treats the sebaceous glands forcing them to stop producing natural oils for the skin or reducing the quantity of the oil produced. this treatment is generally directed to the sebaceous glands on the facial skin.

What Is The Overall Experience Of Laser Acne Treatment?

Most patients who have undergone laser acne treatment report that during the application of the laser light they experience a rubber band type of experience where the laser is applied. If you are uncomfortable with the sensation the doctor will apply some local anesthetic cream on the treated part to dull the sensation. However the end result is a very pleasant.

Nlite Acne Scar Removal

A scar left behind by an attack of acne can be with you for the rest of your life, but if you are lucky you will have treated acne well in time to avoid scarring. However, many people are not so lucky so thank the stars for technology that now offers them a way to get rid of scars caused by acne. Though the medicinal creams and treatments are not too successful when it comes to removing scars there are ways that skin specialists and doctors are able to remove scars and reinstate the glow to the skin with technology.

The advancements in technology have been astounding, especially so with medical technology. Acne scar removal through laser treatment is a developing procedure and is growing popular by the day. Nite Acne scar removal technology was introduced as late as in 2003. This is a technology that can permanently remove acne scars by as much as 100 percent.

The heat energy emitted by the laser equipment is directed at the affected glands and helps tone down the excretion that is the cause of acne. Mostly a painless treatment, the Nite laser acne treatment is not meant for all acne patients. Some patents respond to acne laser treatment better than others. Though laser treatment effectively removes acne scars it may not be 100% satisfactory for all acne patients, tough someone with lesser than 80% scar removal will rarely be found, if at all.

All acne scar removal laser sessions rarely last over an hour with the treatment requiring 4 sittings at 30 day intervals. This treatment kills the bacteria present in the cells of the skin with the intense yellow light that penetrates deep within the skin cells and kills the infection. The treatment also can be used to treat the cells that are producing excess oils leading the disorder called acne. Over 50% of acne affected skin was cured completely within three to six weeks of treatment with Nite acne scar removal technology. Such is the effectiveness of the treatment.

Nite Laser Treatment for acne removal is a dream come true for all those suffering from acne and the scars caused by the disorder. Being a very new treatment the cost is not as yet definite and is expected to stabilize very soon the world over once the technology is easily available everywhere and much more affordable too. In the mean time acne scar removal through the one and only means - laser treatment - can be expected to cost the sky. People with the money to try the treatment are ready to give it a try, such is the suffering many experience from acne

infections. It may be early days yet say many skin experts, but there have been no adverse reports of this treatment, which is being compared to laser hair removal technology - it may well be along the same lines with the same after effects - skin irritation for a couple of weeks.

Acne Treatments For Black Skin

No matter what the color of your skin, acne can be just as menacing to anyone. This is a skin disorder that strikes fear into the hearts of teenagers and adults alike. Yes, adults have finally awoken to the fact that acne is not a skin disorder that only strikes teenagers. The sooner one realized they may have acne the better the chances are of curing the disorder.

Acne does not look for any particular skin color to infect. The disease treats one and all alike, let there be no doubt all are equal for acne and all will find acne just as difficult to cure once it consolidates its position within the cells of the skin it chooses to infect. So white skinned individuals are not the only ones who suffer from acne, black skinned people are just as susceptible, though acne may not have been noticed due to the color of the infection blending into the skin.

Now there is not need for black skinned people to despair as there is a cure for all types of acne. Different individuals respond differently to acne treatments and so the time required for acne to be completely cured varies from individual to individual and so patience it the main requirement and ingredient for a proper cure for the disorder. There are many treatments to choose from and the best treatment for you will be chosen by your doctor. Remember that there is no difference in acne treatments for black skin or white skin. Acne is acne and there are treatments that work effectively on every skin. It just takes time that is all.

Prevention is better than cure

Nothing can be nearer the truth. It is better to be on the look out for any signs of acne. At the very onset attack those pink pimples with the proper treatment - cleanliness. Wash the affected area at least thrice a day with a mild unperfumed skin cleaner. A harsh soap used to clean the affected area will remove all traces of oil from the skin. Though removal of oil is necessary some amount of oil is required for healthy skin. Never apply oily substances to the skin if you notice any signs of acne. A rule of thumb is to discard the use of any product that contains isopropyl alcohol. This substance dries the skin and forces the glands to produce excessive oil that is the main contributing factor to acne infections.

How To Win Your War Against Acne

Natural acne treatments

Nature has hidden many cures for human disorders. Some fruits and vegetables have natural substances that are known to cure acne completely. Some of these are cucumber, lemon, tea tree oil, oats, lime, honey, orange, tomatoes and turmeric. A paste made from any of these fruits or vegetables can be applied to the affected area as a face mask for half an hour every day and rinsed with luke warm water will help in destroying the bacteria causing acne and also remove the excessive oil being produced by the skin. This is a very enjoyable home remedy for acne infected black skin - or any type of skin.

Acne Treatment: What To Do When Acne Strikes

Acne is a dreaded skin disorder that no teen will like to think about. This on disorder that can prove to be the bane of existence for any one who suffers form it. Acne has a way of disrupting ones social life and hindering any form of entertainment because of the very ugly nature of the disease. The unfortunate aspect of this skin disorder is that it cannot be avoided, if it has to strike you will get it irrespective of your race, cast or creed. If you are fortunate enough you might get away with a tiny red bump on your face or if your are less fortunate you might have the disorder all over your body - and once you get it seems like it is going to stay with you for life.

Home Treatment For Acne

If you notice that you have some innocent looking bumps on your face, it could be the beginning of acne. From the moment you notice the bumps you should be very particular to keep the area very clean and free from oil and grease.. This can be achieved by washing the affected area frequently like thrice a day with a mild skin cleaner that must NOT be perfumed. Harsh soaps and cleaners will leave the face completely free from oils that is also not recommended.

After cleaning your face pat the skin dry taking care never to rub the skin with a towel or tissue. Rubbing the affected area will only cause redness and irritation. A good home cleansing routine should be carried out thrice a day with benzoil peroxide. A generous amount of the cleaning agent on the tip of the finger can be applied on some areas of the face. After dabbing the cleanser on the face it can be spread gently to cover the entire face. Moisturizer can be applied about fifteen minutes later without ever washing the benzoyl peroxide of the face.

Some more points to take note of

•   No matter how tempting the feeling of a good squeeze might be, never squeeze an acne pimple. Do not even scratch it.

•   As a rule never touch an acne affected area of your skin. If you have to touch the pimples, do so with a tissue not even with a handkerchief.

How To Win Your War Against Acne

Acne treatment is known to take millions of years, so have you should be prepared to spend a few patient weeks or a couple of months at least. Patience, patience, patience.

Acne Treatment - Orally

Oral acne treatment is another effective way to cure acne. This treatment requires the patient swallow tiny medicated pills that hopefully will resolve the issue. However, these pills may have to be changed frequently in order for the skin specialist to decide which is the best combination of antibiotics for the treatment of acne. This treatment varies from person to person. Contraceptive pills have been known to treat acne in women and very effectively too. A certain pill known as Diane has a certain ingredient 'cyproterone acetate' that is known to clear acne effectively.

Adult Acne: The Three Main Sources

Being the dreaded disorder of the skin that it is, acne has forced many an individual, teenager and adult alike to carry the scar and burden of infection for many years without any sign of letting up. In face it can recur if not treated properly. Many a teenager has discovered that after years of suffering from acne and finally getting rid of the disorder they wake up years later to find red bumps on their face. these bumps begin to spread quickly and they never know the reason why acne returned to torment them once again.

People are beginning to realize that adult acne is a disorder that is more common than perceived in the past. It is believed that more than five percent of acne patients are adults well past their twentieth year. Some of them are nearer their fortieth year. Adult acne is not only confined to the facial areas of the skin but can also make its presence known on the back, neck and on the hands as well.

There are three main sources of acne, or rather three reasons why some individuals are more prone to acne than others. We list here three of the main reasons for acne to strike any one. This may be a start for you to understand the treatment and prevention of acne.

Hormones: the first source of acne

Hormones may sometimes seem to be worth more trouble than they are worth. A little shift in the aging process of an individual and the hormones go into over drive causing glands al over the place to react. Some of these glands take their hormonal instructions a little too seriously and begin to excrete more oil into the skin than is actually required. Experts are still groping in the dark as to why hormonal changes cause these oil glands to flood the system with their oily substance. Fortunately enough they have managed to produce a cure for this cause of acne by controlling the hormonal shifts. One common way for treating adult acne in women is the contraceptive pill that controls hormones in their system.

In the process of groping in the dark and deciding (or discovering) that contraceptive pills cure acne in women, scientists have come to the conclusion that he substance 'retinoids' are the reason that clogged pores get cleared, in effect clearing acne as well.

Stress: Second source of Acne

Another great way to get yourself a bout of acne is to really stress yourself out mentally. Now don't go about blaming yourself for the stress in your life the world is quite good at producing many reasons for your stress. There are bill to be paid, children to take care of, your teenager daughters acne problem and what not. Keep up the stress levels and you are surely going to get an acne treat. Stress in the system triggers the secretion of a hormone called cortisol. This cortisol causes the body to secrets a whole army of hormones that result in the cells developing infections. So if you find your face developing some stress bumps, relax, get rid of the stress, go on a vacation.

Many people who discover the zits on their skin will do well to de-stress, bathe thrice a day, relax and unwind. It may be a good idea to run like the devil to your skin specialist too.

Those Beauty Products: Source Number Three

People tend to over do it with the grooming products in the market. Acne is mainly caused by excessively oily skin and applying creams and skin applicants like foundation etc will only speed them on their way to an attack of acne. These products block pores in the skin and prevent the natural cleansing process. The accumulation of oils within the pores attract bacteria that develops into acne. It is advisable to use products that are noncomedogenic that are oil free this is especially true to your moisturizer.

Treating Acne Using Tea Tree Oil

Acne is a growing skin disorder the world over with more and more people getting this dreaded skin disease. The number of adults being affected by this disease of the skin is growing by alarming numbers, perhaps this population of adults affected by acne was always there and it is only now that they are acknowledging that they have acne and need to deal with it. Acne is an inflammatory eruption on the skin and can occur on the face, the most common place for this disorder to be sighted, as well as the back of the neck, arms and the back.

People find this common skin disorder very difficult to treat at the best of time; however, there are people that can rid themselves of acne in no time at all, like a few weeks, while in more people acne can last many tormenting years. The longer one has to live with acne the greater the risks of having to live with the scars acne leaves behind - for a lifetime. Depending on the person some acne products might suit them and some products might not. It is really a trial and error system to determining how to get rid of acne. Then again there are the tried and tested ways that guarantee to rid one of acne or at least reduce it to a great extent.

It all depends on the type of skin affected by acne. Some skin types respond best to medication and some simply reject the treatment outright and these people have to resort to special technical procedures such as Nite acne laser treatment. The medical fraternity is choc-a-bloc with treatments for acne, some resort to herbal medication such as skin applicants or drugs, while there are others who advocate the use of laser treatment for a permanent cure.

It is best to determine the toxicity of the skin before resorting to any treatment of acne. If your toxicity levels are low then you may be able to cure your acne problem with a few researched herbal applicants such as tree tea oil. This is a proven method that has no side effects and leaves a patient very satisfied.

In a recent research publication tea tree oils were assessed for their ability to treat acne and were rated on a scale of 0 to 10 0 being the best result and 10 as a potential threat to the skin. Australian tea tree oil turned up with a result of 0.01 which was the highest and means that it was the best way to treat acne. The treatment preparation is quite easy; one just has to add 2 drops of the tea tree oil to the acne affected area with a piece of cotton wool. Treat a small area at a time as opposed to the whole acne affected face at a time.

How To Win Your War Against Acne

Acne can also be treated with:

1. Desert Essence Blemish Oil (rated 3.8)
2. Doctor Burt's Herbal Blemish Stick with Tea Tree Oil (rated 3.9)
3. Burt's Bees Healthy Treatment Parsley Blemish Stick with Willowbark. (rated 3.9)

Cystic Acne - Causes And Treatment

Cystic acne, as the name suggests, is acne that has grown into a cyst under the skin and is believed to be the worst kind of acne any person can contract. In this form of acne small nodules form under the skin and slowly harden into cysts that are quite painful. Make no mistake, this form of acne must not be treated by self medication at home, it seriously calls for medical attention, and fast. Treatment for cystic acne could last for months or years.

The most common treatment for cystic acne is a drug known as 'Accutane'. This is an oral medication usually prescribed to be taken twice a day for 20 weeks. Accutane acts on the oil producing glands in the skin and reduces the output of oil marginally. In turn this prevents the pores in the skin from clogging reducing the formation of pimples and other skin eruptions. The existing pimples and cysts are also given time to heal as the irritation is vastly reduced due to less oil in the skin.

Accutane also reduces shedding of skin cells and brings down the stickiness levels of the follicles the main culprits in the development of cystic acne. Accutone has a few advantages and these are:

1. Its ability to prevent extensive scarring of the patient suffering from acne.
2. Somewhere between 1 to 20 weeks of treatment acne is visibly reduced and in some patients acne is completely cured.

The disadvantage of accutone is that once one starts the treatment they must go through with the whole course of the treatment. Stop the treatment mid way and acne will return with a vengeance. Apart from this there are other disadvantages of taking this treatment and these must be considered before starting the treatment.

The disadvantages are:

1. Expensive drug. Can burn a hole in your pocket.
2. Decreased blood cholesterol, triglyceride and lipid levels.
3. Abnormal liver enzymes.
4. Dry mouth, nose, and skin

5. Skin itching and painful muscles.
6. Inflammation of the mucous membrane of the eyes and mouth.

Perhaps the most serious side effect of accutone is possible birth defects. This is why women taking the treatment must take a pregnancy test every month in order to stop the treatment should they conceive. If you are on Accutone and notice any of these side-effects mentioned above notify your doctor immediately in order to take preventive measures. Luckily though, the side-effects diminish and disappear after the drug is stopped.

How To Treat Back Acne

Teens and adults the world over are facing a growing occurrence of this skin disorder called acne. As people flock to the medical fraternity for treatment of this growing skin menace a lot of information about acne is becoming available for analysts and scientists who are working hard to come up with better ways to effectively treat the condition. Most people think of acne as a condition that affects the face, this is probably because acne is mostly seen on the face of a person. The truth is that acne can also affect the back, neck chest and hands of a person as well.

Just as it is common to the face acne also erupts on the back and chest and seldom on the neck of a patient. When acne develops on he back it is very difficult to treat mostly because of the toughness of the skin on the back. There are different products to treat acne on the back for this reason. Another reason for the difficulty of treating acne on the back is that the skin on the back is in constant contact with some clothing at all times of the day and night. This irritates the condition making it harder to treat.

The cause of acne is the secretion of excessive skin oils by the cells of the skin causing the pores of the skin to clog and develop pustules and pimples. As prevention is better than cure it is advisable to prevent acne anywhere rather than have to treat the condition. Especially so when it occurs on the back.

It is important to stick to a regular cleansing routine. Keep cleaning the affected area at least three times a day. You should use a cleanser and a moisturizing lotion. Glycolic acid is a good enough cleaner and works well because it does not leave the skin too dry while it does remove the excessive oils from the skin. While keeping to the cleansing routine one must try to access what is irritating the acne on the back. There are a few things that could aggravate an acne condition on the back:

1. Wearing heavy back packs causing abrasion on the shoulders and back.
2. Certain types of clothing you wear could also irritate acne.
3. Sun and heat could be affecting the condition.
4. Rain or sweat could be another irritant.

How To Win Your War Against Acne

If you regularly wear a heavy backpack and you notice an aggravated state of your condition try to switch to a shoulder bag or hand bag for some time and look out for improvements in the condition. If there is none then the irritation is caused by some other condition. Perhaps certain types of clothing or materials may not be suiting your acne condition. Experiment by changing your style of clothes. Wear more airy clothing to facilitate better circulation of air over the affected area. Wear cotton clothes that are non-abrasive. Keep out of the sun as much as possible. Radiation from the sun is a known irritant of acne. Rain and sweat are also known to be the two main culprits that aggravate acne on the back so try to keep your back as dry as possible.

Laser Treatments To Help Cure Acne

Acne is becoming a scourge that is growing more and more difficult to live with. With the skin condition spreading to more adults as well as teenagers there are many different types of treatments that have been used to treat this condition. Some of the treatments have been successful and some fail drastically. The secret is in discovering which treatment will work best with which type of skin.

For the lucky few acne can be treated with applicants and drugs that are available over the counter, but then there are the less fortunate who try to treat acne with these self-medication products and they are not so successful. In the meantime vital time is lost and acne consolidates itself and becomes very difficult to remove, in the event leaving behind ugly acne scars that may last a life time.

It is best to let a doctor decide which treatment is best for acne. Some doctors will recommend laser treatment as the best way to treat acne at the outset. This is because laser acne treatment is a very fast way to rid oneself of acne with little or no time for the condition to get rooted to the skin making treatment more difficult.

Erbium laser treatment for acne scarring is fast gaining popularity with the medical fraternity the world over. It is a technique that is being recommended by many doctors for the treatment of acne as it prevents scarring. Erbium is also known to effectively heal scars left behind by acne.

While laser is a very good treatment for acne it can be a bit on the expensive side so science has come up with an alternative treatment for acne during the active period of the disorder. This is a treatment that involves the use of aluminum hydroxide crystals that are used as an abrasive to remove layers of the skin. The abrasion removes the dead layers of the skin that assist in the spread of acne and cause a hindrance to the treatment of the disorder. Though this treatment is used only with the most severe forms of acne it is seldom used on acne that threatens to spread over the area. Aluminum hydroxide crystals are best used in areas such as the back and neck as these places are difficult to reach and need effective and fast treatment.

Acne treatment requires a lot of time and patience for any form of treatment before a person can visibly see the results. Laser treatment for acne scarring is the fastest and the most effective

How To Win Your War Against Acne

way to rid one of acne and acne scars. Abrasive methods such as the use of aluminum hydroxide crystals are good for shallow scarring and not the deep forms of acne scars. It is best to resort to laser treatment for more severe acne scarring for a permanent and effective solution.

The True Cause Of Acne

Acne has been known to occur in the healthiest and most hygienic of people any where in the world. So what causes acne? Is it the environment? The water we use? The food we eat? Or is it some form of allergy? The answer is possible a combination of all.

There is no knowing when or where acne will strike anyone. People of all ages have been affected by this dreaded skin disorder that just does not seem to go away, and if it does go there is no guarantee that it will stay away. That acne was a condition of teenaged skin is a bygone belief of yesteryear, people aged well over 40 have contracted acne and have been stuck with the disorder for years. So acne is definitely not choosy about age cast or creed.

Then what causes acne?

There are cells within the skin that secret natural oils for the nourishment of the hair follicles in the skin in general. These glands are the main culprits that cause acne in individuals. The severity of the attack depends on the habits and the type of skin of the person. The oil secreted by the glands clog the pores in the skin, which lead to infection and accumulation of pus. This is acne that is very difficult to heal.

The kind of food you eat, the place you stay and the way you look after your skin all play a vital role in deciding your risk level of contracting acne. A hot humid climate will lead to a very oily skin. This is the very first indication that must put one on the alert and aversive action must be taken if one does not want to develop acne.

A good way to go about this to maintain a good cleansing routing for the skin. Do not be fooled for a moment that acne only attacks the facial skin. You should give your chest, arms, neck and back equal importance. Wash your face at least twice a day with a facial cleanser such as glycolic acid. This cleanser does not leave the skin dry but leaves behind enough oil to nourish the skin. Never use an oily substance to clean the skin as oil is the natural culprit that clogs the pores leading to acne in the first place. Also never dry the skin completely.

Take care of your back at least once a day along with your neck, shoulders and arms as acne also strikes these places as well. When you have finished the cleansing routine use a good skin moisturizer to replenish the moisture in the skin. This may sound very tiresome but it is necessary if you have signs of developing acne.

Acne is more prevalent in adolescents as they go through a very rough phase of life with their hormones becoming very active during this part of their life. Adolescents experience many eruptions on the skin and at most times these eruptions change into acne. Testosterone is the main culprit causing acne. Make no mistake, testosterone is a hormone found in females as well as males, it is not purely a male hormone.

Stress is another culprit that causes acne so take some time off to meditate and de-stress yourself. It is important to control stress if you want your acne treatment to be effective. Stress produces toxic substances that can cause extra oily secretions that clog pores leading to acne. So clean your skin, and relax then let your acne treatment work for you.

Understanding The Different Types Of Acne

Pimples on the skin are formed the same way only some of them take a course for the worse and develop into what we commonly know of as acne. Pimples develop differently on various people, and so does the medication or treatment react differently to them. Acne occurs mainly when a hair follicle becomes infected. A hair follicle is basically a hair root and acne is formed when this follicle gets clogged with oil and a 'comedo' is formed. The clogging of the hair follicle is caused by excessive oils secreted by the follicle.

As the secretion of oil increases and the follicle gets even more clogged the comedo grows leading to inflammation of the skin near the follicle. Thus a pimple is formed. This pimple may remain under the skin or break through as a bump. There are many categories of acne and each type requires a different type of treatment. Some types of acne and their corresponding treatments are covered here.

First of all we have the non-inflammatory acne. This is what is commonly referred to as a 'whitehead'. This is actually a closed comedo and occurs when the clogged air follicle remains just beneath the skin. You may have noticed a small white bump no larger than a pencil tip just under the skin. This is what we are referring to as a white head. There is nothing to worry about white heads. Just remove them with some hot water and cotton. Never try to squeeze them out. Some steam over the face can help remove white heads quite easily. Then apply some oil free moisturizer after removing the white heads.

When the comedo changes to an open comedo, it turns into a blackhead. This occurs when the white head is pushed through the surface of the skin sue to enlargement of the clogging of the follicle. Do not mistake the blackhead for dirt, it is not so. The darkness of the blackhead comes from concentration of melanin in the skin, the pigment that gives the skin its dark color. Blackheads are an inflammatory form of acne.

The papule, which is a tiny pinkish bump on the surface of the skin, is the mildest kind of acne. These are very sensitive to touch and are a step between non-inflammatory acne and inflammatory acne. You then have pustules that are also small, round lesions. However, unlike papules they clearly contain pus, a sign of infection. The yellowish center of the reddish bump is an indication of pus. Though they do not contain serious amounts of bacteria they do get inflamed due to irritation caused by sebum components.

We then have the very painful nodular or cystic form of acne. These are lesions that are filled with pus and occur deep under the skin. Cystic acne develops when the contents of the infected hair follicle spills over and infects the surrounding tissue and the immune system of the body reacts producing pus. This kind of acne can last for weeks or months developing into cysts that are known to leave very deep scars that are permanent in nature.

Understanding the cause of your acne is an important step in preventing the spreads of the condition and the proper treatment that needs to be followed. It's called getting to the root of the problem.

Using Topical Products To Help Treat Acne

There are many kinds of medications that may be used for the treatment of acne. These are both prescription drugs as well as over the counter kind of products. While antibiotics are the common treatment for acne almost all treatment for all kinds of acne starts with a topical application. Topical products for acne are available over the counter and are applied directly to the affected area.

Topical products kill the bacteria on and under the skin reducing the chances of acne to spread making treatment of acne easier. Topical products assist in keeping the pores of the skin open and maintain the breath ability of the skin. These topical products for acne treatment have been around for a number of years and are available in both allopathic as well as herbal forms.

When shopping for antibiotic topical treatments for acne Clindaamycin is a topical antibiotic that is the most commonly available and the most effective too. Clindaamycin can be obtained in lotion, solution or even gel formulations at 1% strength. It is required to be applied at least twice a day to the infected parts of the skin. Though the skin reacts to the treatment quite well some patients of acne have been known to develop a rash or irritation and treatment has to be stopped. So if irritation occurs consult your doctor for alternative treatments.

Tetracycline is another topical treatment that is fast gaining ground for the treatment of acne. Tetracycline is an oral treatment at most times but is also available in the various topical treatment forms such as lotions, solutions and other applicants. Tetracycline consists of sulfur and sodium extracts and so is known to cause allergic attacks in people sensitive to the drug. Tetracycline is also known to cause a yellow pigmentation of the part that it is applied to possibly due to the sulfur content so the topical application. The side effects occur even if the treatment is taken orally.

Metronidazol is a topical treatment that is available in gel form and is a very effective treatment for a kind of acne that is caused by rosaces. The treatment is required to be applied at least twice daily and does not cause any serious side effects. Many people respond favorably and fast to this kind of treatment though it does cause irritation in some people.

How To Win Your War Against Acne

However it is always advisable to consult your doctor about the best treatment for your acne problem instead of experimenting with over the counter drugs and wasting vital time, time that may well be used to rid you of your disorder and prevent it from consolidating, making it harder to cure.

<u>Ways To Treat And Prevent Acne Scarring</u>

The physical as well as the psychological effects of acne scarring are a difficult condition to deal with for adults as well as for teenagers alike. Perhaps it is more so for teenagers than adults. The medical fraternity are finding it very difficult to understand, more so treat, acne scarring. Why does it have such a long lasting effect? And why is it so difficult to treat? Perhaps we will never know - however doctors have turned to technology to remove acne scars rather than treat it with medications.

Various kinds of acne leave different kinds of acne scars. There is good news though; acne scars can be effectively and permanently treated. Doctors also advise a proper acne treatment that needs to be carried out on a daily basis by the affected individual to prevent the return of the scourge.

The first step in the treatment of acne is to understand the type of skin of the affected person, the kind of acne that needs to be treated and the best treatment for the kind of acne being treated. Acne scarring and the corresponding treatment varied from individual to individual, mainly depending on the kind of skin being treated. Doctors find it difficult to understand what skin type will be affected by acne and to what extent will the skin scar. Understanding this condition is important for the effective treatment of any form of acne.

It is a common consensus that acne must be treated as early as possible in order to treat the condition most effectively and prevent permanent scarring. Acne is not expected to be an overnight procedure. Acne treatment lasts weeks and sometimes years depending on the severity of the condition. This is shy it is important to treat the condition before it consolidates and becomes hard to cure. Many people treat acne as and when it appears and takes preventive measures; however some people find it hard to rid themselves of this ugly mess of pimples and expert help is called for.

The crux of the matter is to prevent inflammation to occur if you want to prevent acne scarring. Remember never to irritate an acne infected area; irritation will surely lead to acne scarring. If you are prone to scarring from acne it is best to consult a skin specialist at the next outbreak of pimples on you skin. Remember early treatment is the secret to prevent acne scarring.

How To Win Your War Against Acne

Acne scars are of two types. Those scars caused by the loss of skin tissue and those caused by formation of skin tissue. The scars that are formed by excessive tissue formation are known as 'kelloids' known as hypertrophc scars to the medical world. The term 'hypertrophy' refers to any enlargement of growth on any tissue. This kind of scarring is caused by extra deposits of collagen in skin tissue. This substance is produced when the skin reacts to an injury and over production of it leads to scarring though this king of scar fades over time.

Scars formed when tissue is lost are very much like scars formed by an attack of chickenpox. These are very common scars and equally hard or rather impossible to treat.

The best way to prevent acne scarring is to prevent the disorder itself. So seek medical help at the earliest when you notice those infamous pinkish bumps on your skin.

What You Should Know Before Taking Accutane

Accutane is a prescription drug for the treatment of very severe infections of acne and is usually resorted to as a last medicinal resort for the treatment of the dreaded skin condition. The kinds of acne that are generally treated with accutane are cystic acne known also as nodular acne.

Understanding The Cause Of Acne

Sometimes, in certain conditions excessive oils are secreted by the glands in the skin and these oils lodge in the hair follicles in the skin and clog the pores of the skin where the hair grown out of. This leads to inflammation of the follicle and the surrounding tissue that result in pimples, which may grow into cystic nodules filled with pus that is tender to the touch. Sometimes the treatment of these cysts requires a physician to drain them of the accumulated pus cells.

Cystic acne is known to last for months even a few years as it is one of the more severe kinds of acne. It is only when the treatment resorted to fails to produce results that doctors resort to the use of accutane as a treatment for cystic or persistent acne. The doctor must, however educate the patient on the side effects of the use of accutane while treating acne. Sometimes a physician will ask a patient to sign a form stating that you understand the side effects of the use of the drug and that you consent to the treatment.

Perhaps the most outstanding side effect of the use of accutane is the birth defects that can possibly occur in the fetus of a pregnant woman taking the drug. Accutane may even be the cause of a miscarriage during pregnancy. Still born babies are common when a pregnant woman resorts to accutane as a treatment for acne. So, if you are pregnant NEVER take accutane as a treatment. If you are not pregnant, doctors require you to undergo a pregnancy test every month if he is treating you for acne with accutane.

Patients of acne being treated with accutane have been known to develop suicidal tendencies as well. The symptoms include:

1. Mood swings
2. Anxiety
3. Depression
4. Irritability

How To Win Your War Against Acne

5. Becoming a recluse

6. Loss of sleep or Excessive sleep

7. Weight loss or gain

8. Loss of appetite or gain of it.

And these are just some of the effects of the use of Accutane. Then is it really beneficial to use accutane at all? You decide.

Accutane must be resorted to as a last resort for acne treatment. Because acne and acne scarring can be a very heavy burden for people to carry due to the loss of social activity and psychological stress associated with the disorder and when nothing else seems to work it may be the last choice for the physician but let it be the last choice of the physician.

Acne Control The Natural Way: 8 Ways To Say Goodbye To Acne

People who want to prevent acne often spend large sums trying to do so. But, they don't have to! There are several natural and inexpensive methods for getting rid of those embarrassing acne breakouts. In addition, these methods can help prevent sudden outbreaks of acne from occurring. Here's some help for those suffering from acne.

Defining Acne

In most cases, genetic predisposition determines the type and severity of acne breakouts. Acne is caused by a combination of hormone activity and natural sebaceous activity under the surface of the skin. Sebaceous, or oil, glands secrete sebum whose purpose is to keep the skin soft and flexible and it is vitally important to healthy maintenance of the skin. A lack of sebum causes dryness, rough skin and even cracks and splits. However, hormone activity combined with diet and other factors, can stimulate the sebaceous glands to produce more natural oils than is needed. This excess can block the pores of the skin, leading to blackheads and a localized infection that we commonly call pimples. Acne breakouts normally occur on the face, neck, back, chest and shoulders which are the most visible areas of the body and is where the sebum glands are most densely saturated.

While individual genetics have been shown to play a significant role in the development of acne, social factors such as daily routines and diet are also major players in causing outbreaks. Genetics may not be subject to change but an individual suffering from acne need not feel powerless or hopeless when it comes to treating their acne. Some simple changes in diet and routine has an enormous impact on controlling and eliminating acne.

Simple Natural Changes to Eliminate Acne

The following is a list of several suggestions for dealing with and eliminating acne:

1. The most important thing to do is probably the easiest, drink LOTS of water. Water flushes toxins from the body and also aids in the creation of natural skin oils and moisture. The better

hydrated a person is the less need for the creation of additional skin oils by the sebaceous glands.

2. Consume at least four to five servings of fresh fruit and vegetables every day. Nutrition science has shown that the natural amino acids in fruits and vegetables are important in the formation and regulation of sebum. Poor nutrition, or a diet heavy in oils, dairy products and fats, leads to more severe acne outbreaks.

3. Try rose water for facial cleansing. Using a clean cotton ball dipped in rose water, moisturize and clean the face and other areas prone to breakouts two to three times daily. Rose water is a natural antiseptic that doesn't strip the skin of natural oils.

4. Avoid using soaps and alcohol-containing products for cleansing. These strip the skin of its natural oils. Harsh cleansers stimulate the skin to produce more sebum to keep the skin moisturized, opening the door to more acne outbreaks.

5. Make-up may also cause acne outbreaks because it blocks the surface pores of the skin. In addition, some types of make-up cause drying of the skin. This stimulates the glands to secrete more sebum to compensate for the drying of surface oils. Choose cosmetics that are natural and do not contain alcohol or petroleum based products. Also, use a natural moisturizer to keep skin soft and pliable without encouraging sebum production. Contrary to popular belief, good quality moisturizers do NOT cause acne and may actually help to lessen outbreaks.

6. At the first sign of an outbreak, apply ice to the area to lessen the appearance of redness and irritation. Use a little rose water to cleanse the area, and pat a little cornstarch or baking soda mixed with water over the area. This will soothe, draw out the infection and ease the discomfort of the outbreak.

7. Cucumber is an inexpensive and effective acne control treatment when used as a mask. Blend it with a little water in a blender until a smooth paste is formed, and pat over the face and other affected areas. Leave it on for approximately 30 minutes and then rinse of with warm water. Cucumber has been shown to be a good acne treatment that refreshes the skin without damaging it.

8. Find out if you have any food allergies. Acne is sometimes the body's way of letting you know that you are allergic to something you are eating. Mild to moderate allergies to cow's milk and milk products, grains, gluten, chocolate and other foods considered to be a normal part of diet can lead to acne outbreaks. A simple way to test for a food allergy is: if you suspect you may be allergic to something, eliminate it from your diet for a few days. If your acne and your general health begins to improve it would be a good idea to discuss the matter with your doctor. A simple allergy test will let you know if you are sensitive to a certain food or food group.

Natural Advantages of Natural Acne treatments

The quest to cure acne has spawned a huge treatment industry. Consumer markets are flooded with products all claiming to eliminate acne, and its often an expensive proposition when trying to choose the best out of this sea of curatives. Unfortunately, many of the products sold to prevent acne often make it worse instead of better. For the wise shopper, natural methods should be the first choice but whether you have tried all the other methods or none of them, its never too late to try the simple, natural methods mentioned in the list above. They are both time and money saving. They will improve your overall health and vitality, and they aren't going to cause the situation to get worse instead of better. So what are you waiting for? A natural cure for your acne is as near as your cupboard or local grocery store!

Oral Acne Medication Options

What causes acne?

When puberty begins, young people begin to experience a wide variety of developmental physical, physiological and emotional changes. The obvious physical changes include beard and muscle development in young males, and young females, with the onset of menses, also start to develop breasts and wider hips. In addition, the normal progressions toward adulthood produce rapid hormone changes frequently causing mood swings and the often embarrassing side effect of Acne Vulgaris.

More commonly known as just simply acne, breakouts or pimples, Acne Vulgaris is caused by an overproduction of the natural skin oil glands. When this excess oil combines with dead skin cells and surface dust, it forms hardened blockages in the ducts leading to the surface of the skin-these are usually called blackheads or whiteheads. Sometimes these blockages produce a localized infection, which manifests as pimples or Acne breakouts just under the surface of the skin. Of course, there are other factors which contribute to the development of Acne breakouts, including diet and genetics, but dermatologists have a great many options available to them for its treatment.

Medical research and breakthroughs

The treatment of Acne has become a multi-million dollar industry. Although Acne may seem very superficial and irrelevant in comparison to many other diseases, its effects on the emotional and spiritual wellbeing of adolescents can have far reaching consequences. The scars left by acne is one of the leading causes of low self-esteem among young adults, and has long reaching effects even for adults. Because of this, dermatologists and medical researchers are constantly working toward the development of better treatment options.

Unfortunately, there is no "magic bullet" in the treatment of Acne Vulgaris because there are many different factors that contribute to its development. However, medical practitioners have been employing several different oral medications for its treatment. Some of these have undesirable side effects, and some cannot be used under certain conditions (such as during pregnancy or before a specific age) but they are often effective in controlling Acne.

Examples of commonly prescribed medications and their effects

The following is a list of commonly prescribed medications for the treatment of Acne. While these treatments have positive outcomes for many users, there are side effects which should be considered when taking them. In addition, no one drug will work for everybody, so sometimes an Acne sufferer may have to try several treatment options. It must be noted that this list is neither exhaustive nor completely comprehensive but is designed as an overview of currently available treatment options.

Antibiotic Acne Medication: Taken orally, various antibiotic medications have been employed in the treatment of acne. Research has shown that many antibiotics ameliorate Acne and are often prescribed for persistent, moderate-to-severe acne. As with all these medications, they should be administered only by a qualified physician.

Cortiscosteroids: This potent antibiotic treatment should only be prescribed for very severe cases of acne, and should only be taken for short periods of time. The metabolic side-effects of steroids have been well-documented and if taken in large quantities, or for long periods of time, may have long-term effects on the reproductive capabilities of young people. As a result, they are not recommended for most cases of acne treatment.

Tetracycline: Tetracycline has been the most commonly prescribed acne treatment for many years. It has had good results for moderate-to-severe acne. The usual dosages range from 500 to 1000 mg per day, and dosage is decreased as the skin condition improves. Tetracycline has been associated with decreased bone development and teeth staining, and therefore it is not appropriate for children under the age of eight. Due to its effects on bone development, it is also not an appropriate choice for pregnant or nursing women. Other common side effects include increased sun sensitivity, diarrhea and nausea.

Minocycline and Doxycycline: Derived from Tetracycline, research suggests that these drugs may be more effective in the treatment of Acne. Both drugs have higher concentrations in the tissues and have been associated with more effective and more rapid improvements in visible Acne. Doxycycline may cause sore throats or heart burn and must be taken with large amounts of water. Minocycline has been associated with drug induced lupus symptoms but is the least likely of the Cycline drugs to induce photosensitivity. However, skin pigmentation problems do occur with both these medications. The higher concentrations of both drugs in the tissues may

also lead to liver reactions. Neither is appropriate for use in young children or for pregnant or nursing women.

Erythromycin: Available in both oral and topical applications, is a safer alternative for pregnant women and young children. It has the advantage antibacterial and anti-inflammatory treatment results, reducing both the cause and the effects of acne. Its oral form is easy to use but may cause some gastrointestinal upset. It is also a good alternative for those who are allergic to penicillin and the cyclines.

Isotretinoin: Derived from Retinoid A, this antibiotic is a revolutionary new treatment that has been shown to be highly effective in the treatment of severe and treatment resistant Acne. Clinical trials have shown it to be beneficial for all forms of Acne, but there are many side affects attributed to Isotretinoin. These include severe effects such as birth defects, excessive dryness of mucous membranes and the skin, depression, inflammatory bowel disease and erectile dysfunction. There are several other milder effects which should be thoroughly discussed with a physician before this drug is prescribed. In addition, there is disagreement among medical practitioners concerning the dosage levels needed for optimum effects and the long term effects are still under investigation.

3 Popular Myths About Acne

No one likes it, but almost everyone will experience it. For some people, it is a constant source of embarrassment and even low-self esteem. What is it? Acne!

Acne pimples appear on the face, neck, and body and are usually small red bumps although for some people these bumps can become cysts. Acne also tends to afflict everyone, to some degree, regardless of race or gender. Usually appearing in adolescence, it is almost an accepted rite of passage into adulthood because it is so common among teenagers. Acne is caused by increased hormonal activity within the skin's oil glands or the sebaceous glands. The extra secretions of oil, combined with dead skin cells and surface dirt, leads to clogged pores and outbreaks of lesions, which we call pimples, blemishes or acne. Acne commonly occurs in the neck, face, back, shoulders and chest because the body's sebaceous glands are more densely distributed here.

So What Determines The Extent and Severity Of Each Case Of Acne?

There are many factors which contribute to acne. For example, there are hereditary components which affect the severity of an individual's acne. Simply put, if you have a parent who has suffered from a severe case of acne, the chances that you will also have severe acne are increased. But there are also dietary and sociological factors that contribute to the development of acne, which if changed or eliminated, may prevent an outbreak of severe acne. Because of the many contributing factors, acne myths have proliferated over the years.

Acne Myth Number 1

Scrubbing and washing the face often will prevent acne. While dirt may contribute to the formation of blackheads leading to pimples, many people believe that washing your face three or more times a day, or hard scrubbing of the face and skin can prevent acne. Face washing should be done gently, using a mild facial scrub or exfoliant only twice a day. Frequent washing can actually irritate acne breakouts and it strips the skin of its natural oils. This not only makes the skin dry, but can lead to the sebaceous glands increasing oil production to protect the skin surface. Also, scrubbing can cause inflammations. Gentle cleansing, using the lightest possible touch, is best for all-round skin protection.

Acne Myth Number 2

Fried food, overeating, and chocolate, causes acne to develop. Diets heavy in fat do have an effect on the body's sebaceous glands, but science has shown that moderate consumption of fried foods will not cause acne to get worse. In fact, some oils are necessary for the healthy maintenance of the human body and the "acid mantle" that keeps skin moist and supple. In addition, a seeming connection between certain foods such as chocolate and acne may be due to food allergy rather than to the food itself. The notion that any particular food always causes acne is quite false, though.

Acne Myth Number 3

Daily stress will cause breakouts of acne. Routine, daily stress is not considered to be a cause of acne. Severe stress has been shown to have detrimental effects upon many of the body's systems but its connection to acne breakouts has not been clearly established. More research is needed in this area before anything conclusive can be formulated. One caveat, though, stress medications may have a side-effect of contributing to acne, but if so, this should be discussed with a physician as an alternative medication may not have this effect. In general though, stress is a normal part of life and is not regarded as a major contributor to acne.

6 Acne Skin Care Tips

A significant number of people of all ages suffer from skin problems such as rashes, blemishes, blackheads and acne. Commonly developing during puberty, acne usually occurs during a time of life when the individual is the most vulnerable and socially insecure. This makes acne not only a physical condition but sometimes an emotional and/or psychological one. Acne can shatter an individual's confidence. Acne breakouts are the result of excessive secretions of oil from glands under the skin, leading to a buildup that blocks the ducts leading to the skin's surface. Acne primarily affects the face, chest, back and upper arms. Some people continue to suffer from acne related skin infections for many years past their adolescence, although it usually diminishes during early adulthood. There is no definite way to determine when acne breakouts will stop.

Acne is frustrating for many people because it is unpredictable and sometimes seems out-of-control. Breakouts have been attributed to several factors, including diet, heredity and genetics, vitamin deficiencies and stress. Since the exact causes acne are still unknown and there isn't any measure available to prevent it. The best defense is a good acne skin care regimen which ameliorates and controls acne breakouts. For more severe types of acne, such as cystic acne, a dermatologist should be consulted since medical treatments are advisable to prevent or lessen scarring, but for milder forms of acne there are many options available.

Six General Tips For Living With Acne

1. Washing twice a day, using mild cleansers and gentle movements is the best acne skin care regimen. Gentle cleansing removes excess oils, dirt, and pollutants which contribute to the development of blemishes. Strong detergents, harsh scrubbing, and harsh facial scrubbers irritate the skin and may contribute to inflammation and breakouts. Also, its best to avoid opening the blemishes since it may spread the infection over the skin. Squeezing pimples may also cause them to burst under the skin infecting other skin pores as a result, dermatologists strongly advise against doing this. Shampooing regularly also helps to prevent acne by keeping the natural oils from hair off of the skin surface.

How To Win Your War Against Acne

2. Astringents may be helpful for very oily skin but should be avoided for other skin types. Choose astringents and other topical applications carefully, if they are too strong it may cause more oil production and irritation.

3. For men, shaving should be done carefully in order to avoid irritating or spreading acne. Choose a safety razor that is right for you by testing out a few. Soften beards by first washing the face and neck with mild soap and warm water; then apply a shaving cream. Use care in selecting the shaving cream because many contain ingredients such as menthol that may irritate your acne. Use a sharp razor and shave lightly to avoid cuts and rupturing blemishes.

4. Exposing your skin for a while to the sun may help to erase blemishes at the skin surface. The natural vitamin D in sunlight has been shown to improve skin quality. Nevertheless, care should be taken to avoid excess sun exposure which leads to premature aging, dryness and sunburn, and the development of skin cancer. Some prescription medications also cause photo-sensitivity. Discuss with your physician whether mild sun exposure may help with your individual case.

5. Individuals with acne should use oil free cosmetic products. Many cosmetics contain fatty acids that may be harmful to acne prone individuals. Select good quality cosmetics but be aware that some "oil free" products may be drying to the skin. Look for organic or acne-related skin care products to lessen the impact of cosmetics upon acne. Keep in mind that topical applications for acne treatment, such as some Benzoyl peroxide products, may react with the facial cosmetics.

6. It is best to consult a dermatologist before applying any acne skin care product. Particularly for serious cases of acne infection, treatment by a dermatologist is advisable to keep acne under control and to prevent breakouts. Observing proper acne skin care is important especially for younger individuals. Blemishes and rashes tend to heal faster when a person is younger but severe acne cases should be properly taken care of to prevent scarring. A healthy diet and lifestyle will also lessen the effects of acne.

Coping With Adult Acne

For many years the skin condition, Acne, has been associated with adolescence and those "difficult" teen years. Since most adolescents experience some degree of acne, it has long been assumed that hormone levels directly impact acne, and goes away when a person reaches maturity and hormone levels balance out. And it is true that hormonal activity does play a role in the development and severity of acne. Hormones promote the manufacturing of sebum or oil; excess oil blocks skin ducts and pores causing acne. However, many times acne problems continue on after a person becomes an adult, and sometimes these problems increase during adulthood and the child-bearing years. Adult acne is simply not as uncommon as has been previously supposed.

Adult acne can be just as frustrating and embarrassing as adolescent acne, perhaps even more so. There are many social, emotional and psychological effects of acne, which, together with the physical symptoms, contribute to a lower self-esteem. Those who suffer from adult acne may withdraw from social situations fearing that their condition makes them conspicuous. They may suffer from a lack of confidence or embarrassment due to scarring and breakouts.

The Causes And Treatment Of Adult Acne

Adult acne was thought, until recently, to be a rather uncommon occurrence. This is because fewer adults were willing to seek treatment, leading to a lower instance of reported cases. Many adults are embarrassed that they have a condition which is usually considered an adolescent's disease, are afraid of the opinions of others, concerned about their personal image, and are reluctant to seek professional help as a result. Consequently, although adult acne is fairly common, it has not received much attention up to now. There are many factors leading to the development of adult acne, treatment should be based upon a case-by-case basis. A dermatologist should be consulted and an individual skin care regime determined upon. Pre-emptive skin care treatments can preclude harsh, aggressive, and sometimes even dangerous treatments once the flare-ups have gotten out of control. Adult acne and its symptoms are better managed through proper, preventative acne control methods.

As more information about adult acne has become available, the instances of reported cases have been on the rise. Attention and better information dissemination has caused more and

How To Win Your War Against Acne

more adult sufferers to realize that they are not isolated. Women of child-bearing age and even into their late thirties and forties frequently suffer from acne for much the same reason as teens: hormonal activity. This is also true for male sufferers. More recognition of this problem has led to better treatment options for adult sufferers. There are many treatments available to relieve adult acne, some over-the-counter and others by prescription. A dermatologist can help you to determine what treatments are right for you.

Another aspect of adult acne that makes it difficult for adults is the scarring caused by acne. Aging skin is thinner and not as resilient as that of an adolescent, which isn't as much of a concern for young adults as it is for older sufferers. Prolonged acne can cause scars that are deeper and more visible. Since adults are just as concerned about their appearance as younger people may be, the emotional effects of acne may have a deeper impact upon adult sufferers. Good quality moisturizers and other skin treatments can lessen the effects of acne scarring.

Whatever the type, acne treatment is vital to the health and wellbeing of adult acne sufferers. Treatment also has emotional benefits because it allows an adult to feel that they are taking action to improve their situation. In some cases, a combination of therapy and treatment may be advisable. In any event, treatments are now available that can smooth the road to recovery for adult acne sufferers.

How To Determine Your Skin Type

The type of skin that you have plays an important role in how acne will affect you and also in how you should treat it. Different skin types need different types of treatments in order to effectively handle acne. One size definitely does not fit all when it comes to acne skin care.

There are four basic types of skin, oily, normal, dry, or combination skin, a combination of two of them. Combination skin may be normal-to-oily or normal-to-dry. For each type, a different skin care regimen is needed. Skin types also change over time, skin that may have been combination normal/oily may become more normal or dry as the skin ages. Changes in skin requires adjust of skin care routines to maintain a healthful appearance.

Five Questions To Ask Yourself

First, start with some basic questions in order to determine your skin type. The answers to these questions will help you to decide what type of skin you have.

1. How frequent are your breakouts?
2. Do you have blackheads?
3. Do you have large pores?
4. How does the skin feel after it has been washed with soap and water?
5. Are there facial lines?

The answers to these questions help determine the type of care your skin will require to look its freshest.

Basic Descriptions of Skin Types

Each skin type is determined by several factors such as the amount of oil produced, texture, and the frequency of acne breakouts. Skin tones often seem to coincide with certain types of skin, but skin tone is not a determining factor in what type of skin you may have. Quite fair skin may also be oily, while dark tones may be dry. Therefore, skin color is not a good metric to use when determining what type of skin you may have.

How To Win Your War Against Acne

People with dry skin usually have few breakouts and seldom experience blackheads. The reason for this is that excess oil blockages are what form blackheads, and dry skin is not prone to excess oil. This generally means that acne breakouts are rare for this skin type, although other problems may exist. Dry skin generally has few if any visible pores, and the skin will feel tight and/or dry after cleansing. Those with dry skin are usually fair-skinned and often develop facial lines early in life. This skin type may sunburn very quickly.

People with normal skin and with combination skin suffer occasional breakouts, with mild-to-moderate blackheads that occur for the most part in the "t-zone." The t-zone is the area which runs across the forehead and down the nose and mouth area, it also includes the chin. Pores are often larger and more noticeable in the t-zone area but are usually not as large as those that appear in oily skin. The skin may feel dry and tight immediately after cleansing but will soon feel more lubricated. The skin tone for normal skin usually is fair to medium, and a few early lines may appear around the eyes. This skin type usually will sunburn when first exposed to the sun, but then will tan. Prolonged sun exposure can produce temporary dry skin conditions.

Oily skin is characterized by more frequent breakouts and the presence of comdones or blackheads. The pores are enlarged and visible. After washing the face quickly becomes oily, the nose and forehead quite rapidly growing shiny due to increased oil production. The skin tone is frequently olive or dark. Facial lines are not very prevalent with this type of skin; oily skin tends to be resist aging longer than the other skin types. Therefore, over the long term, oily skin stays youthful for a longer period of time than the drier types of skin. Oily skin rarely burns when exposed to the sun and usually tans easily.

A Final Word

Determining what type of skin you have should enable you to make better choices when it comes to skin care products. There are numerous products on the market that are designed to improve skin quality. For improving your acne, choose products that won't cause further problems for you by basing your choices upon the type of skin that you have. Adjust your skin care regimen as your skin changes in order to be on top of your acne problem.

Natural Acne Treatment

Let's face it, almost everyone has acne occasionally. It's not because you are eating fried foods or chocolate. It's not because of stress or a lack of personal hygiene. Acne is caused by impurities in the skin and body. Thus, internal cleansing may be the way to get rid of acne or to at least keep it under control. Topical medications and oral antibiotics may not clear up breakouts because they only target one or two of the causes of acne or just treat the symptoms. This can mean that a lot of different treatments may be required to handle a specific case of acne. And many treatments can have very undesirable side effects.

Natural methods of controlling acne go by various names such as Herbal, alternative, and holistic remedies. However it's referred to, natural treatment is becoming one of the most popular forms of therapy for many diseases, including the treatment of acne. More and more people are viewing illnesses as a systemic problem, indicating that the body itself is out of balance and needs to be refortified.

Four Herbal Medicines That Help Cure Acne

Natural acne treatments work best for moderate cases of acne. They are designed to cleanse the system internally of toxins that contribute to the development of acne breakouts. The advantages of natural acne treatment are that it not only attacks the visible symptoms but treats the internal causes of the acne. Natural methods usually involve modifications in the diet because it focuses on cleansing the internal organs. These types of cures utilize herbs that nourish and heal vital organs and also aid in internal cleansing.

Herbal preparations and topical preparations that have been shown to be effective for the treatment of acne are:

1. Olive leaf extract-believed to strengthen the liver.
2. Herbal cortisone-mimics prescription cortisone as an effective treatment for acne without side effects.
3. Jing Huang Gao - a Chinese herbal cream for removing and preventing blemishes.
4. Tea Tree Oil-used topically, considered as effective as benzoyl peroxide treatments.

How Does Natural Acne Treatment Work?

Herbal acne remedies target the liver because it is the organ that cleans the blood of hormones. Hormones have been shown to influence acne but they also insure the body functions properly. When hormones are being over-produced it can lead to acne breakouts. Herbal treatments contain many plant nutrients that are rich in vitamins and minerals which the body needs to stay healthy and to function at peak efficiency. There has been no evidence to show that natural medicines have any negative side effects when used for treating acne and they are available without a prescription. In addition, herbal medicines may kill the fungi that weaken the liver. Many herbal treatments are designed to be taken seasonally, such as those that are intended to cleanse the colon and flush body toxins. Others may be taken daily as a regular supplement or used as a topical ointment.

A healthy liver functions much better, and does a better job of removing excess toxins and hormones from the system. This prevents the toxins from finding their way out of the body through the skin's pores which leads to acne breakouts. The advantages of natural treatments are clear and certainly should be given a trial when trying to eliminate acne.

Should You Use Makeup To Cover Up Your Acne?

Acne may leave the skin blemished, scarred, red, and blotchy. Sometimes, the scars left by acne will lighten over time but many times they do not. For many people, covering the symptoms of acne is a priority, particularly for those who work with the public. Sometimes acne scars are relatively easy to conceal because they are caused by less severe cases of acne, or acne that was treated early in its onset. Deep scarring, caused by more intensive acne, usually requires some form of cosmetic surgery to remove because they are much harder to conceal with make-up and other cosmetic products. For light scarring, make-up can save the expense involved in medical removal of the scars by a dermatologist or cosmetic surgeon. It is also helpful for those forms of acne that are minor or only localized breakouts. In these cases, makeup products can enhance the look of your skin, giving it a smooth, even complexion, and a fresh, bright appearance.

What Makeup Products Are Right For You

When deciding upon the makeup products to use for covering acne and its scars, avoid products that are "comedonic" (products which may clog pores), creating blackheads which can lead to acne breakouts. Products containing oils and petroleum products are more likely to cause blackheads and should be avoided. Instead, choose non-comedonic formulations that do not contain these additives. Check the labels carefully. While there is a wide range of products that are marketed for acne, a lot of consumers find that when correctly applied "ordinary" makeup will often serve their purposes. Don't be afraid to experiment until you find the right products for your skin's needs. Also, your dermatologist may sell high quality products designed for this purpose, ask for samples if these are of interest to you.

If you have a history of sensitive, problem skin, select a make-up that is light, not oily, and non-comedonic. There are numerous powders and foundations for sensitive skin on the market. Consumers who have especially oily skin should consider a tinted powder, which is modifier that can help control the oil and reduce shininess. Sometimes, medicated products may be right for you, particularly if you are wearing it for long periods of times. Be wary of those products that are designed to "treat" acne as many of them may be very drying to the skin. As previously mentioned, don't be afraid to experiment with the products you are considering. Many products are available in sample forms, which allow you to test them out.

How To Win Your War Against Acne

Take care when selecting a powder or a foundation that you select a product that is not harmful to your skin. Don't use products that make your face peel, itch, or burn. These kinds of products are damaging your skin and only adding to its problems. Also, when using make-up to hide acne scars, don't use a tint that is too dark or too light. Choose shades that match your skin's tone, and apply it evenly over the surface of your skin. Don't concentrate larger amounts on blemishes; this will only attract the eye to that area. If foundation alone isn't sufficient to cover the acne, you might consider a concealer. Concealer is available in many forms and is frequently used to cover blemishes to help reduce the visibility of acne, as well as dark eye circles and other skin blemishes. Again, you may need to experiment to find the product that is right for you.

Remember, acne scars often lighten over time, and the day may come when you won't need to worry about covering them anymore. However, make-up may help to reduce the impact of acne for you until that day.

Understanding Teen Acne

Acne is very common for teenagers, and often impacts more than just their physical appearance. It can also negatively affect their self-image and self confidence, making them reluctant to participate in social activities and sports. Acne is caused by increased hormonal activity within the skin's sebaceous (commonly called oil) glands. It affects teenagers because adolescence is a time of increased hormonal changes. The extra secretions of oil, combined with dead skin cells and surface dirt, leads to clogged pores and outbreaks of lesions, which we call pimples, blemishes or acne. Acne commonly occurs in the neck, face, back, shoulders and chest because the body's sebaceous glands are more densely distributed here.   However, help is available to combat the effects of acne.

Two Common Mistakes In The Treatment Of Acne

Acne has little to do with diet, except in cases of food allergies, or by too much facial washing. These are two common myths often associated with this condition. Too much facial cleansing can cause the skin to become dry and irritated, aggravating and inflaming existing acne breakouts, but it does not cause more acne to form. If acne pimples are ruptured by cleansing that is too rough or by harsh products the infection may be spread over a wider area.

In addition, it is not advisable to pinch or pop acne pimples. Pinching can drive the bacteria that cause acne deeper into the skin, creating more or deeper pimples under the surface. Rupturing pimples allows the infection to escape onto the surface of the skin, clogging and infecting surrounding pores. Although it has been a common practice, it really isn't a good idea.

Five Truths About Acne Treatment

1. Since adolescents usually produce more skin oil than adults, it is important to cleanse twice a day with a mild cleanser that won't dry or inflame the skin. This cleanses excess dirt and oil away from the skin. It is also important to keep the skin properly hydrated and moisturized. Oily skin doesn't mean that the skin is properly moisturized. Attempting to dry oily skin by harsh cleansing often causes the glands to work overtime to re-hydrate the skin. Using a light moisturizer helps to prevent the secretion of excess skin oils.

How To Win Your War Against Acne

2. Facial cleansing has the added benefit of preventing more acne from forming because it removes those agents that cause acne: excess oil, dead skin cells, and surface dirt. Since the goal of acne treatment is prevention, a good skin care regimen is the best place to start.

3. While exfoliants are a good idea, choose one that is gentle to the skin and which has small grains. Smaller grains are not as harsh, aren't as likely to scratch the surface, and won't aggravate acne. They gently remove dead skin cells, freshening and beautifying the skin. Also, don't scrub your skin; use light, circular movements to exfoliate without damaging the skin.

4. Avoid products that contain substantial amounts of alcohol. Alcohol has a drying effect upon the skin, causing it to produce more oil to compensate for that moisture which has been stripped away. If using a toner, choose one that contains no alcohol.

5. Choose make-up products wisely. Avoid those products that may have caused or contributed to past breakouts, and select only those that won't clog pores and create blackheads. Never go to sleep with make-up on, always wash it off before going to bed.

Although no one can combat their physiology entirely, acne can be controlled by a good skin care regimen. In cases of persistent, severe acne, or where cystic acne may exist, the best course is to consult a physician. There are a lot of medications that can treat acne; it is not something that you must "suffer through" alone. Finding a solution is the best way to improve self-esteem.

Understanding The Psychological Effects Of Acne

Acne is probably the most prevalent skin condition among both adults and adolescents. The physical appearance is not the only thing affected by acne; many people suffer psychological effects as well. Often they will avoid social interactions and events because of the insecurity they feel. Appearance, in modern society, has assumed monumental social importance. How we look often affects other people's perceptions and evaluations of us, and more importantly, our estimation of ourselves. For teenaged sufferers in particular, the stress created by this social pressure can cause low self-esteem and low self-image that continue to affect people long after they have reached adulthood. Social acceptance during the teen years is more important than at any other time of life. So what happens if a person has a physically altering condition like as acne?

Why Acne Has Such A Negative Psychological Impact

During the teen years, people begin developing a strong sense of self. It is the time when individuality begins to surface and also a time when social conformity is the most important. There is no other time in life when social acceptance is of such paramount importance as it is during adolescence. Studies have shown that the psychological effects of acne may lead to depression, social anxiety and withdrawal, and eating disorders. When a teen suffers from a disfiguring case of acne, his or her sense of self is profoundly impacted and it doesn't just go away. Many adults labor with the psychological effects of acne, feeling ugly, conspicuous, and undesirable long after they have left adolescence.

Another factor that may affect self-esteem for adolescents is the misconception that acne is caused by a lack of hygiene. While this isn't true, it may contribute to the anxiety felt in social situations. Acne is primarily linked to hormonal activity, and not to personal hygiene, but this perception may play into self-image issues for both adolescents and adults.

What Can Be Done To Help Prevent Acne-related Psychological And Emotional Damage

The first step toward improving self-image is to understand what causes acne, and to take the necessary steps to prevent acne breakouts. Minor cases of acne may be handled by a proper skin care regimen, and sometimes, by eliminating diet-related causes. Food allergies have

How To Win Your War Against Acne

been shown to sometimes increase acne. Severe acne usually requires medical intervention to treat it. Whichever way you choose to go, being proactive in the treatment of acne is always best, it increases self-esteem.

Occasionally, as previously mentioned, diet plays a role in acne breakouts although it is generally believed to affect adults more than adolescents. There may be foods that influence acne due to allergies or individual sensitivity to certain food groups. For those who may feel that their acne gets worse when they consume a certain food, try avoiding it for several days. If the acne improves during that time, you may wish to avoid that food or to consult a physician for an allergy test. If the acne is related to a food allergy, the allergy will not go away over time. It may require permanent dietary changes.

Topical concealers, available over-the-counter or by prescription, may be utilized to hide the scarring caused by acne. Some dermatologists carry make-up and other skin care items that are designed to both heal and hide acne. Whichever method works best, don't be afraid to try a few topical applications but avoid those that contain petroleum products or heavy oils. Acne is caused by blocked pores so heavy concealers may actually increase the problem.

For those that may be suffering from anxiety or depression, it is always best to talk these matters over with a physician. There may be other factors besides acne that are causing these conditions; a doctor is best equipped to diagnose and treat those. Don't be afraid to seek help for your acne or for any emotional problems that it may be causing you.

<u>Water As A Natural Acne Remedy</u>

Many products have been created to treat acne. There are over-the-counter topical creams and ointments, cleansers, and medicated pads; and medicine and ointments prescribed by a physician. Natural remedies have been increasing in popularity for treating many common ailments, acne included. However one of the most preferred, and possibly surprising, treatment options is: water.

Water is one of the best remedies available for acne. Your body is about 70% water, and requires constant replenishment to remain healthy. The skin is the largest organ in the human body, and like the rest of the body it must be properly hydrated to fulfill its functions. Consuming plenty of water will keep the skin looking and feeling healthy. Healthy skin cells promote a healthy body. In addition, drinking lots of water helps to flush toxins from the body. Deep in your skin, water is a crucial component, providing the basis for a healthy, youthful complexion. Though very little water is stored in the outer layers of your skin, this moisture is important and is constantly removed by exposure to the environment.

Sun and wind can dry your skin, causing irritation and inflammation. When this happens, acne can become worse, perpetuating the acne cycle. While irritation doesn't necessarily cause acne, it can worsen the problem. Drinking lots of fresh water helps to eliminate the environmental factors that lead to acne inflammations.

Perhaps one of the most common myths is that oily skin does not need moisture. This is not true. Just because skin is oily, does not mean it is moisturized. By cleansing the skin, you are wiping away excess oil, and my moisturizing it, you are helping it remain smooth and decreasing your chances for irritation.

Properly hydrating the skin not only promotes and stimulates cell growth, but also helps the other organs of the bodywork together. Water is also the primary transporter of nutrients throughout your body. If not enough water is consumed, toxins can build up causing breakouts. Water flushes these toxins out. By drinking at least 8 glasses of water a day, you are flushing out the toxins that would normally escape through the pores of your skin, and in turn, preventing acne breakouts.

How To Win Your War Against Acne

In addition, proper cleansing using mild cleansers and water, aid in replenishing the skin's vitality. It is a myth that acne prone or oily skin types do not need moisturizers. In fact, cleansing removes some of the surface moisture and a light moisturizer will help to replenish this loss. It also combats the environmental effects on the skin. When this layer of natural moisture is removed, the skin's gland will begin to secrete additional oils to replace it, leading to more acne breakouts. Always, use a light moisturizer after cleansing in order to prevent this from happening.

Though water is not the only natural remedy for the skin, it is the most important. Without an adequate supply of water your body cannot clear waste products which stack up in the cells and your blood. Doctors advise us to drink six to eight eight-ounce glasses of water a day. While this sounds like a lot of water, think of what it can do for your body. In addition to improving skin tone and texture, it can stimulate cell growth, improve the functions of body organs, and reduce the effects of acne.

What Causes Blackheads And How Are They Treated

Comedones, more commonly known as blackheads, are one of the most common causes of acne, particularly for those who have oily skin. It is caused by excess oils that have accumulated in the sebaceous gland's duct. Generally, when acne vulgaris begins, its starts as blackheads and whiteheads. The difference between them is that a blackhead, or open comedo, is open at the surface of the skin. A whitehead, or closed comedo, is hardening of the oil in a closed environment under the surface of the skin. Both of them contribute to the formation of pimples and acne breakouts.

At one time, it was believed that comedones formed because of too little cleansing, but it has been shown that they are created by a combination of oil, dust and dead skin cells within the pore itself. The "black" appearance of a comedone is caused by oxidization acting on the oil, melanin (color pigments in the skin cells) and keratin in dead skin cells clogging the pores which creates their dark appearance.

Treating Blackheads

The best way to prevent blackheads is to alleviate their cause: excess oil and dead skin cells. Use gentle cleansing products that are designed to treat comedones. Avoid using products that contain alcohol, mineral oil or petroleum-based additives as these are harsh and actually may make the problem worse instead of better. Stripping the skin of its natural acid mantle (emollients and oils produced by the skin) actually stimulates the glands to produce more oil, perpetuating an acne cycle. Products containing natural oils and ingredients are less likely to block pores, and usually are more gentle to the skin.

A gentle exfoliant to remove dead skin cells may be used on a daily basis. However, most dermatologists recommend the use of these products twice per week, to avoid irritating the skin. All exfoliants should be used in a gentle manner, don't scrub or use hard rubbing movements when using them.

Avoid hard squeezing to remove the blackheads. This may cause further irritation resulting in pimples since it may force part of the blockage deeper into the skin. It is best to employ gentle methods of removal, such as blackhead removal strips and products designed to dry them up.

How To Win Your War Against Acne

Although is a longer method to take than quickly squeezing them out, it is better for the skin in the long run because it avoids scarring.

Occasionally, diet plays a role in acne breakouts although it is generally believed to affect adults more than adolescents. There may be foods that influence acne due to allergies or individual sensitivity to certain food groups. Most physicians maintain that proper diet helps decrease oil production, provides moisture to the skin, and helps facilitate the growth of new and healthy skin cells.

As previously mentioned, blackheads are usually prevalent in oily skin types, but they can occur in dry, normal and combination skin, although with less frequency. Skin care products should be chosen carefully because they are essential to preventing and healing acne and blackhead breakouts. A healthy diet and lots of water are also key to maintaining a fresh, clean complexion. There are many over-the-counter products for treating blackheads as well as prescription medications available from your dermatologist. If blackheads occur, eliminate them gently using mild cleansing products and topical creams designed to dry them up.

When To Seek Medical Attention For Your Acne

For both adolescents and adults, acne can be an aggravating problem. There are many variations of acne and differing degrees of severity. The physical, emotional and psychological effects can be devastating, affecting an individual 's confidence, self-image and self-esteem for many years. Although several of the milder types of acne respond well to over-the-counter treatment products, more severe forms require medical attention. Acne care is vitally important regardless of the type, but it is just as vital to know when a case of acne requires a dermatologist to treat it.

Three Reasons To Consult A Physician

The decision to see a physician or dermatologist about your acne should take into account several things:

1.   Is your acne causing you emotional difficulties?
2.   How severe your outbreaks are.
3.   If your skin seems to be scarring when the lesions heal.

There are several more reasons why it may be wise to seek professional help with your acne but these three comprise most of them. Severe acne may leave permanent scars; seeking medical help early on may help to reduce the effects of scarring. The best way to prevent scarring is, of course, to prevent acne from occurring in the first place. The right skin care regimen and possible dietary changes, are needed to control acne breakouts.

Recent studies have shown that food sensitivities may contribute to the formation of acne, such as allergies to wheat, dairy and certain fruits. One such study has shown that women consuming three or more glasses of milk per day were 22% more likely to have acne breakouts than women consuming only one glass of milk per day. This may be due to the hormones present in fresh dairy products, but some dermatologists are recommending that their patients with cystic acne avoid mild products and use alternative sources of calcium intake. The type of acne and skin type plays an important role in how acne is best treated.

How To Win Your War Against Acne

If you have cystic acne, also known as nodulocystic acne, it must be treated by a physician. Do not try to treat it yourself because it can cause very painful lesions and scarring of the face, neck, back and shoulders. Cystic acne resembles small bumps or tumors, blackheads may not be present with it, sometimes the lesions fill with a combination of blood and pus, cystic pimples may involve more than one pore, and they are very deep within the skin layers. This type of acne should be treated by a dermatologist as quickly as possible, in addition, some dietary changes may be needed to decrease the outbreaks of this type of acne.

Emotional distress, such as severe anxiety, depression or social reclusiveness, are also good reasons to seek professional assistance. Severe acne sufferers feel helpless to control the situation particularly for adults due to the notion that acne should clear up once a person becomes an adult. Acne scarring has long term effects, often affecting a person's choice of occupation, social interactions and dress. A medical professional can help to restore a person's self confidence as well as helping clear up the acne.

For men, sever acne can shaving difficult. Shaving irritates pimples and lesions, may irritate existing scars and lead to further outbreaks of acne. A good razor, shaving creams and other products help to reduce the irritation and inflammation of acne, but a medical professional can also prescribe creams and medications to eliminate it.

It may be a good idea to visit a dermatologist at the outset of acne, even if you aren't sure that it is a severe form of acne. Medical advice can help in the choice of skin care products, provide assistance regarding acne care and daily routines even if prescription medications aren't required. In severe cases of acne, a physician is indispensable to help reduce the effects, treat the cause and prevent future outbreaks.

This Product Is Brought To You By

DAVID A OSEI